DONOR

DONOR

HOW ONE GIRL'S DEATH GAVE LIFE TO OTHERS

John Pekkanen

LITTLE, BROWN AND COMPANY   BOSTON · TORONTO

FIRST EDITION

*Some of the material in this book was previously
published in* The Washingtonian.

LIBRARY OF CONGRESS CATALOGING-IN-PUBLICATION DATA

Pekkanen, John, 1939–
    Donor, how one girl's death gave life to others.
    1. Donation of organs, tissues, etc. — Social aspects.
2. Organ donors — United States — Biography. I. Title.
RD129.5.P45   1986   362.1'795 [B]   85-23157
ISBN 0-316-69792-3

Designed by Jeanne Abboud

*Published simultaneously in Canada
by Little, Brown & Company (Canada) Limited*

PRINTED IN THE UNITED STATES OF AMERICA

For John Boswell, Jack Limpert,
and, always, my wife, Lynn. Thanks
for being there.

AUTHOR'S NOTE

This is a true story. For reasons of
privacy, the names of the donor family and
the recipients have been changed, as have
some other identifying details. However,
the names of all the medical people, as well
as the medical institutions, are real, and the
events portrayed in this book occurred as I
have related them.

ACKNOWLEDGMENTS

I was able to write this story because of the trust a number of people placed in me. They gave me their time, allowed me to be a part of their lives, and I am in their debt. Jo Leslie was an invaluable help throughout. She opened many doors, and her candor permitted me to understand the difficult and valuable work she did. Others I want to single out are Fran Danella and Bob Grant, Jo's coworkers at the Maryland Organ Procurement Center; Melville Williams, M.D., head of the kidney transplant program at The Johns Hopkins Hospital; Jimmy Light, M.D., and Kathy Oddenino, R.N., at Walter Reed Army Medical Center; Kenneth Kenyon, M.D., at the Massachusetts Eye and Ear Infirmary; Paul McEnery, M.D., John Noseworthy, M.D., Clark West, M.D., C. Frederic Strife, M.D., and Monica Quinlan, R.N., all of Cincinnati Children's Hospital; Ron Dreffer, Organ Procurement Coordinator in Cincinnati; Betty Irwin, R.N., and Walter Stark, M.D., both of Johns Hopkins; and Michael Lemp, M.D., and Charles Hufnagel, both of Georgetown University.

For other reasons, I must also thank Will and Jessica Davis, good friends, for making me feel welcome during my many visits to Boston; John Boswell, my literary agent, for being a consistent source of support throughout; Jack Limpert, editor of the *Washingtonian*, where this project originated, for his continuing encouragement; Bill Phillips, senior editor at Little,

Brown and Company, for his thorough and thoughtful editing, which made this a stronger book, and also for his encouragement of it; and Barbara Crandall, for carefully typing this manuscript.

I owe a special debt to my wife, Lynn, who helped me with this book, and in life, in ways I cannot begin to express. I also want to tell my three children, Robert, Sarah, and Benjamin, that their love and patience did not go unnoticed, and I also want to thank them for helping me better understand what I was writing about.

Finally, I want to thank the four recipients, their families, and the donor family, for trusting me with their stories and for teaching me so much about the courage and generosity of the human spirit.

~~~~~~~~~~~~~~~~ PART I

THE FIRST
FORTY-EIGHT HOURS

It was a chilly March night. High, rolling clouds gathered in a moonless sky. A front was moving in and there was a feel of rain in the air. The two young girls felt the quickening wind bite against their faces as it gusted through the trees and tall grass of the nearby fields.

Lisa Kelly was small and lithe and moved quickly in the darkness as she and Joanne made their way along the edge of the two-lane country road. They headed toward the shopping mall, less than a mile away. Lisa and Joanne, both high school juniors, were close friends who spent every Saturday night together, at the movies, bowling, partying with friends, or just talking at home.

"Last time we'll have to walk anywhere," Lisa said. "I'm getting my car next week."

"The red one?" Joanne asked.

"Yeah," Lisa answered, "the 'seventy-six Plymouth."

"I can't wait," Joanne shouted over the wind.

Lisa had saved nearly fifteen hundred dollars from her part-time job as a dietitian's helper at a nearby hospital. Earlier that night, she'd rushed home after work and extracted a promise from her father to go the following Monday and buy the car the two of them had picked out. She'd hugged him around the neck and thanked him, and made him a promise of her own: "I'll be a careful driver, you wait and see."

He smiled at her. "I know you will, honey."

She'd hugged him again and was so excited she couldn't finish dinner. She had even passed up homemade apple pie, her favorite dessert.

Lisa and her father were close. Every spring and summer they tended their vegetable garden together, weeding it and picking tomatoes, peas, carrots, and other vegetables as they ripened. They'd recently made plans to raise chickens. Their relationship was so loving no one would have thought that Eugene Kelly was not Lisa's natural father.

When Lisa was very young, she had been abused by her natural parents. Then her skin was jaundiced, clumps of hair were missing, and she had the potbelly of the malnourished.

But at the age of three, Lisa was sent to a new home, and new parents, by a Maryland social service agency. In the Kelly household, she was raised with love and trust, and for years she'd taken the Kelly name and family as her own.

Even as a baby, Lisa was strikingly pretty. Her eyes had always been her most riveting feature, and long ago they had shed their uncertainty. Now at seventeen they were large and blue and glowed with a gentleness that was the essence of Lisa. "Everyone's friend," her mother often said of her, "a real mother confessor." Lisa's skin was soft and clear, and her long blond hair fell in waves alongside her face. Now it tossed as she hurried.

Lisa and Joanne had waited for a ride to the shopping mall, but it never came, so they walked. Lisa had to buy a present for Pamela King's birthday party. It was a little past 8 p.m. and the party had already begun.

"Pam will have a fit with us so late," Lisa said.

"She'd have a fit anyway," Joanne answered, laughing. "Pam couldn't go a day without having a fit."

Lisa smiled. Pam was the type who saw life as an unending

crisis. Lisa had pretty much decided to buy her a record album, probably Fleetwood Mac.

They neared the gas stations and small stores at the intersection where two narrow blacktop roads emerged out of the rural darkness and met. The mall was a couple hundred yards away. Despite the stop signs, and later the traffic light, it was a difficult intersection to get across.

Lisa was dressed in jeans and a light-blue parka with white sleeves she'd bought for a skiing trip earlier in the winter. She was a good skier and wanted to go back again, up to Liberty Hill in Pennsylvania or Blue Knob in Virginia, or maybe to Deep Creek Lake in western Maryland. With a car, she could go anywhere.

Lisa was also wearing heavy wooden clogs that clomped on the pavement. "You sound like a horse," Joanne said.

They approached a stretch of road near the intersection and peered into the darkness at the small rise. Nothing coming. "Let's go," Joanne said, as she darted across the road. Lisa followed.

Headlights suddenly glared from over a small hill; they eemed to come out of nowhere. Both girls bolted. Lisa was usually the faster of the two, but her clogs slowed her down. Joanne made it to the other side. She screamed for Lisa to hurry, but in that last paralyzing instant, as the car skidded, she realized Lisa wouldn't make it. Lisa was only a few feet from the edge of the road when she was struck.

The sounds of terror filled the night air. Joanne sobbed. "Oh God, oh God," she repeated over and over, with her hands squeezed tight against her face. Then came the wail of approaching sirens, the rescue squad, fire trucks, and police. Onlookers collected and spoke in whispers: "Who is it?" In the distance there was a small pinprick of white light in the night sky, then it came closer, and the hard, throbbing sounds of the state police helicopter ambulance grew louder. It hovered, then landed in a nearby parking area. Police and rescue workers struggled for nearly an hour to free Lisa, who had become entangled in the car's damaged front end. Once free, she was placed on a stretcher and wheeled to the helicopter. Intravenous lines were hooked to her, vital signs taken. She remained unconscious.

Now, at a little past 9 P.M., the engine of the helicopter whined faster and faster, the blades smacking against the air. Everyone at the accident scene watched in silence as the chopper kicked up wind and dust, slowly lifted off, and carried Lisa Kelly's small, broken body to Shocktrauma in Baltimore, thirty miles away.

Jo Leslie wrapped the leftover fried chicken in aluminum foil and wedged it into the refrigerator. Then she carried the dinner dishes from the small dining room table to the kitchen. Rick, her boyfriend, helped load them on the dishwasher's racks. She hit the start button on the dishwasher and glanced at the clock. It was close to 10 P.M. She didn't eat late to be fashionable; it had been a long day.

Jo had hazel eyes behind round, caramel-framed glasses, and her light-brown hair was almost shoulder length. Her manner was informal. Her narrow, attractive face was intensely alive, seeming to hold reservoirs of energy. She was joyful, dedicated, and, at times, profanely funny. Her lilting voice still echoed the cadences of her native Tennessee. She was thirty-one and divorced.

For the past several months, Jo, trained as a physician's assistant at the Duke University Medical Center in North Carolina, had been director of the Maryland Organ Procurement Center in Baltimore. Her job was to procure donor organs, a field she'd been in for three years.

She went into the living room, picked up the Saturday *Bal-*

timore Sun she hadn't had time to read yet, and sat down in an easy chair. She took pride in her home, an old dry-cleaning shop when she bought it. She had renovated it, keeping much of the rich, old wood she'd wanted and tearing down the walls she found confining. She had done much of the work herself.

Her two-story home was near Patterson Park, a lively, middle-class neighborhood on Baltimore's east side. A back deck overlooked an alley that was often busy with children playing and neighbors talking. In the spring and summer, she cultivated a small vegetable garden on the deck. It had never borne much fruit, but the labor provided escape from the tensions of her work.

Before she'd turned five pages of the newspaper her beeper sounded. She made a noise somewhere between a sigh and a groan and went to the phone.

"Jo," the familiar voice of the nurse said, "I think you'd better come over here. Looks like we may have one for you."

"What is it?" Jo asked.

"Young girl with a head injury," the nurse said. "Came in by helicopter about twenty minutes ago."

"Be there in a flash," Jo said, hanging up.

She turned to Rick and shrugged. They'd wanted to spend a quiet evening at home, doing nothing.

He shrugged back his understanding; he'd grown accustomed to the sudden changes of plans that were part of Jo's work. They embraced and kissed.

"I'll see you when I see you," Jo told him.

Saturday night traffic was light as Jo's Volkswagen bus bounced and banged over the potholes made by a hard winter. She had grown attached to Baltimore and now thought of it as home. She liked the pace and feel of the city. She drove onto Lombard Street and made two right turns, pulling between a cluster of tall buildings at the rear of Shocktrauma and the University of

7

Maryland Hospital. A blue sign with white lettering read: TRANS-PLANT TEAM EMERGENCY PARKING. It was a little past 10 P.M. She took an elevator to her office on the sixth floor, slipped on a white lab coat, and ran down three flights of stairs to the trauma admitting area. She had walked these corridors often, usually late at night, usually on weekends. That's when most accidents happen. She was the one who decided whether a critically injured person would be a suitable organ donor, and then approached the family to seek permission. It was difficult work and nearly half the time she failed. As sensitively as she approached every family, they often refused out of fear, igno-rance, religious beliefs, or simply because the idea of organ donation appalled them.

If they consented, she then oversaw the many details involved in donation. The organs might go to someone as near as her own hospital or as far away as Europe. Still, it was this first stage, approaching the family, that made her job so difficult.

As she neared the trauma admitting area, she heard the buzz-ing voices of the doctors and nurses and saw the helicopter pilot standing in the hallway. Baltimore's Shocktrauma is one of the best trauma care facilities in the country, a place where medical miracles are performed almost routinely. It is brilliantly lighted; even the green ceramic tile on the walls sparkles. Jo looked up at the lightbox on the wall near the trauma bay entrance. On it was an X ray showing the round, white shape of a human skull. If it were normal, the whiteness would be smooth and unbroken. This one wasn't normal. The whiteness of the bone was intersected with dark lines, running in different directions, like rivers on a distant landscape. Jo knew she was looking at the worst: an eggshell fracture of the skull. It was Lisa Kelly's X ray.

In the middle of the six-bed admitting room, surrounded by defribulator pads, sterile instrument packs, oxygen, and other resuscitation equipment, doctors and nurses worked feverishly

8

over Lisa. She lay motionless. Their voices were sharp and clipped, their hands and eyes moved quickly.

"Give me a CO_2 reading," a doctor demanded.

"Twenty-eight," a nurse answered.

The nurse squeezed a black rubber bag, trying to force more oxygen into Lisa's lungs. Jo watched as the weary, defeated face of a young doctor looked up. He hadn't given up, but his look told Jo that he knew he wasn't going to win this one.

The trauma resuscitation protocol is designed for speed and aggressive overtreatment. You don't quit until it is certain that death is inevitable. Within seconds after Lisa was taken from the helicopter, everything that could revive her was tried, including an array of drugs, additional intravenous lines, hyperventilation, and more. A small catheter had been inserted into her skull to drain off excess fluids, and the air splint on her shattered leg remained as the medical team concentrated on her head injury.

The only good signs were that her pupils were still reactive to light, and her vital signs were stable. But even as they continued to work on Lisa, to exhaust every last avenue of hope, her brain continued to swell, damaging it still more. The minutes passed. There would be no medical miracle for Lisa.

A senior neurosurgeon turned and spoke to Jo, who stood in the doorway. "Looks like she's a candidate for you." His statement was flat and unadorned; it was the language of death.

"When I saw that skull X ray I thought so," Jo said. "Is her family here yet?"

"I heard they're on the way," the doctor answered. "I'll have to talk to them." He flipped what was left of his cigarette butt into an ashtray and took a deep sip from a cup of coffee. He wore the expression of someone with a very painful job to do.

Jo moved closer to Lisa. A nurse pumped up the blood pressure cuff on Lisa's right arm and with a stethoscope listened to an artery near her elbow for the sounds of her pulse.

"One ten over sixty," she announced. Lisa's blood pressure was still normal.

Jo was not immune to seeing people die, and she knew she never would be. She had toughened herself to look at death hard and steady, without blinking. The curtain of doctors parted slightly and Jo saw a young girl who was so delicate she almost looked like a child. She drew in her breath and stepped back. The death of adolescents always hit her hardest. They were just on the edge of life, ready to experience it fully, and the possibility was gone. But the essence of her work was to extract life out of death and seek a standoff between the two ancient enemies. It was work she thought was vital, and she was committed to it. Jo knew nothing could save Lisa Kelly. And as her life slipped away, Lisa was becoming one of medicine's cruel ironies: an ideal candidate for organ donorship.

She was young, with a fatal head injury, and presumably possessed healthy organs. In her death was the possibility of giving life, or sight, to others. Lisa could offer to them a medical miracle that could no longer be offered to herself.

Jo looked down at the small plastic bag at the foot of Lisa's bed. It collected clear urine through a catheter, a sign that Lisa's kidneys were functioning. Jo stepped out into the corridor and over to a coffee pot in a small room. She'd been up very late the night before to receive a kidney that came in from North Carolina. Two long nights, she thought to herself, as she drank black coffee.

She thought about having to meet with Lisa Kelly's family. Emotions were charged and these encounters were unpredictable. The father of a teenage boy once fainted and collapsed in front of her, and the brother of a gunshot victim tried to assault her when she suggested organ donation. And she'd never forget the mother of a sixteen-year-old boy who, high on Quaaludes, played Russian roulette with a .32 caliber pistol, and lost. His mother was beyond consolation.

Jo had no idea how the Kellys would react, or how complicated the night would become.

The Kellys are a country family, large and close-knit. The spreading word of Lisa's accident quickly drew them together. Tommy, the Kellys' twenty-one-year-old son, arrived at his parents' house and picked up his father to drive him to Baltimore. Louise Kelly had already left with Maureen, her married daughter who lived only a few miles away.

It was an hour's drive from the Kelly home to Baltimore. Eugene Kelly, a quiet man in any circumstance, sat mostly silent in the front seat of his son's car. He was nearly sixty, a carpenter. He'd built the snug house in which his family lived. He had powerful, rounded shoulders and meaty hands. Before a heart attack the previous fall, he'd never been ill. In his mind he kept replaying the words of the state trooper who'd come to his door a little after 9 P.M.

"I'm sorry, but I have some bad news for you, sir," the trooper said.

"What is it?"

"Your daughter Lisa has been struck by a car out on Route Four Twenty-one. We've taken her to Shocktrauma in Baltimore, by helicopter."

"How bad's she hurt?" Eugene Kelly asked, his heart racing.

The trooper answered with no expression. "She's still got a pulse."

Those were the words that made hope most difficult. Lisa must be badly hurt if the most the trooper would say was that she still had a pulse.

The roads to Baltimore were hilly and twisting. Sometimes in the distant night sky Eugene Kelly could see the yellow glow of Baltimore's lights above the dark horizon. He thought about dinnertime, just three hours earlier. Lisa had been so excited about getting her car. It was all she'd talked about. Pictures of her face floated in his mind, the little girl, and the young woman. He struggled to hope.

Maureen, always steady, drove her mother toward Baltimore. She was only minutes ahead of her brother and father. Louise Kelly sat in the front seat and dwelled on the irony. She'd thought her real worries would begin the next Monday, when Lisa bought a car.

Maureen, a registered nurse, was worried not only about Lisa, but about her parents, too. She feared the strain this put on her father's heart. She also knew her mother was a deeply emotional woman who was very close to Lisa. In the dim light of the car's interior, she could see her mother moving a handkerchief up to her eyes, and she heard muffled sobs. She reached over to her mother and tried to break the tension.

"She may not even be hurt that badly, Mom," Maureen said. "They probably took her to Shocktrauma just as a precaution. They're doing that a lot now."

Louise Kelly, too, struggled to maintain hope. "I know they took a young boy there about two months ago and I read in the papers they released him the next day."

A rush of thoughts about Lisa came to Louise Kelly. She remembered fourteen years earlier when she first came to know her. Lisa's natural father, a man of limited intelligence, and her emotionally unstable mother had abused her. Custody was taken away from them, and the Kellys were called by the state.

"I have someone for you," the social worker said. "A very troubled three-year-old girl who needs a home."

At the time, the Kellys had three natural children. Donald and Maureen were in high school, and Tommy was beginning elementary school. But there was such an abundance of love in the family that they could care for more children. They had regularly accepted neglected children for foster care, not for the small amount of money the state paid them, but because they saw a need for it.

The social worker explained that the young girl had suffered very disturbing experiences. There once had been some suspicion she was retarded. That was put to rest after she was tested and found to have a normal intelligence. Her big problem now was that she was so frightened it was hard for her to communicate with anyone.

Louise Kelly realized Lisa was in worse shape than other children she'd taken in, and she wanted to talk it over with her family. She needn't have. At dinner that night, they all agreed they wanted to take Lisa.

A week later, Lisa arrived. The signs of neglect were obvious, but the moment Louise Kelly laid eyes on her she knew she wanted to keep her. Lisa haunted her. She baked Lisa a chocolate cake that first day. When Lisa ate it, she dropped a little of it on her dress. She tried frantically to rub it off, to make her dress clean. Louise realized that Lisa must have been punished severely for getting dirty. So she went out to the backyard and sat on the edge of the sandbox. She waited and waited until Lisa came out into the sandbox and began playing.

"Roll around in the dirt all you want," Louise said. "Getting dirty doesn't matter to me."

Lisa played in the sand, but still she wouldn't speak.

When the Kelly children arrived home from school that afternoon, they all gathered around Lisa and made a fuss over her. They talked to her and asked her questions. But Lisa still would not say a word, nor did she smile.

After dinner that night they took her shopping at a nearby department store and when they were driving home, Lisa put her new underpants on her head, as if it were a new hat. They all laughed, but Lisa remained quiet. When they were home they took Lisa's new clothes and laid them out on her bed. They kept telling her that they were her new clothes and finally Lisa spoke her first words.

"Mine?" she asked, pointing to the clothes.

"Yes, that's yours," Louise told her.

For the first time Lisa had spoken to the Kellys, and now she smiled, too.

The three Kelly children made Lisa their little sister in every way. At first Tommy, the youngest, was the only member of the family who understood her, so he became Lisa's "interpreter." The family came to call her the "blonde bombshell."

But it would be months before Lisa would allow any of the Kellys to hug or hold her. And it would be longer before the most obvious effects of her first three years disappeared. But the love and understanding the Kellys gave Lisa won out. The nightmares, tantrums, and crying gave way to laughter; the fun-loving little girl was coaxed out of the frightened child.

Lisa became a favorite of Maureen's, who was sixteen at the time she arrived. Maureen had always wanted a sister, and now, because her parents had given her so much affection, she was able to give it to Lisa. She drove her places, took her to movies, taught her to use makeup, baked cookies with her, and as time went on had sister-to-sister talks with her. To Maureen, Lisa was a sister, as close as blood. Later, after Maureen married, Lisa babysat for Maureen's two small children and often cared for the young foster children the Kellys continued to bring to their home. Lisa seemed to have a special bond with little children.

Two years after they took in Lisa, the Kellys were asked by the social worker if they would take in Lisa's younger sister, Ellen, who had been living in another foster home. They welcomed her. Like Lisa, Ellen was very attractive, but they were different. Lisa was softer, more vulnerable, more trusting. Ellen was stronger and more resilient. Like sisters, they fought, but they also grew very close.

As the years passed, it became apparent that Lisa's natural parents would never be able to care for the two girls. And during those years the attachment between the Kellys and Lisa and

Ellen deepened. There came a time when it seemed Lisa and Ellen had always been Kellys. The Kellys' love for them in return was as absolute as if they had been born into the family. Adoption proceedings were started. By the time both girls entered school, they had their names legally changed to Kelly. The adoption proceedings dragged on for years, but the Kellys persisted. They wanted no one else to take care of these little girls. Lisa and Ellen felt the same. To them, the Kellys were Mom and Dad. Only in the past few weeks were the adoption proceedings drawing to a close. In a few days both Lisa and Ellen would be the legally adopted daughters of Mr. and Mrs. Eugene Kelly.

Maureen wound her way through the unfamiliar streets of Baltimore, looking for Shocktrauma. Louise, clinging to hope, vacillated between thinking the worst and wondering if Lisa would be well enough to go out and buy her car on Monday.

Maureen tried to joke. "Lisa will be fine, but we'll never find our way out of Baltimore." She and her mother laughed nervously.

They arrived at the University of Maryland Hospital and saw a hospital policeman.

"Can you tell me how to get to Shocktrauma?" Maureen asked.

"You here for the little blonde?" he asked. He seemed to be smiling.

"Yes," Maureen answered, and a surge of hope went through them. Why would he smile unless he knew Lisa was going to be all right?

Maureen parked in a small lot and they headed for the fortress of brick, steel, and glass. Bright lights glowed from every window of the six-story building.

Maureen took her mother's hand as they walked in the cold night air. They both felt a tightening in their chest.

Maureen looked around. "This has got to be the way," she said, walking through a set of doors and down a long, empty corridor.

They moved toward a collection of old chairs in a waiting area. Maureen and her mother sat down. In a few minutes, her father and younger brother, Tom, arrived.

"Any news?" they asked.

"Nothing yet," Maureen answered. They all felt cold. A group of people walked past, laughing. How can they laugh? Maureen thought, and then wondered if she'd ever laugh again.

Louise repeated over and over, "There's got to be hope. There's always got to be hope." She sobbed as she spoke.

Maureen knew her mother was on the edge. They continued to wait. Minutes were like hours. Maureen put her arm around her mother. She looked at her father, a face of stoic melancholy. What would this do to him?

Finally, they heard footsteps. The senior neurosurgeon, dressed in a green surgical scrub suit, approached. His face was taut and drawn. It was a face that gave bad news. His voice was soft, but certain.

"I'm sorry," he said. "Your daughter has an irreversible brain injury. There is no hope for her."

"No hope?" Louise asked, her voice breaking. "No hope at all?"

"No," he said. "I'm very sorry."

He stayed to answer questions. How can there be no hope if she's still alive? Couldn't there still be a miracle? Don't these cases sometimes reverse themselves? "No," he kept repeating, "I'm sorry." Their questions ended, and the surgeon left.

Louise and Eugene Kelly sat down, both devastated. Maureen turned toward a corner of the room, squeezed her mother's hand, and wept uncontrollably.

Jo Leslie hurried up a flight of stairs, carrying Lisa's urine sample to the pathology lab on the fifth floor. Time was the enemy. Organs have very limited lives outside the human body: seventy-two hours at most for a kidney, and some medical centers will not accept any more than forty-eight hours old, despite the best efforts to preserve them.

There was another reason to hurry. Despite the modern medical technology now keeping Lisa's body alive and maintaining blood flow to her vital organs, severe brain damage was unpredictable. The brain stem, the center that controls heartbeat, breathing, blood pressure, and other life-giving functions of the body, was being crushed by the pressure of Lisa's swelling brain tissue. Lisa's breathing could stop at any time, and all hope of procuring her organs for others could suddenly be lost. So Jo tried to get the edge on the time she knew would be absorbed by talking to the family, getting an operating room, finding a surgeon, locating potential recipients, and making flight connections. There was little time for her to think in these situations, and that was usually a blessing.

Jo gave the urine sample to a lab technician who would examine it microscopically for telltale clumps of cells. These would signal kidney damage. Other checks had to be made. Jo headed to the Shocktrauma communications center on the fourth floor and called the state police barracks. She reached the trooper who'd investigated Lisa's accident.

After explaining who she was, Jo said, "I have to know if Lisa Kelly's heart ever stopped beating at the scene of the accident." If it had, even for three or four minutes, it could have irreversibly damaged her kidneys.

"Not as far as I know," the trooper answered.

"At no time?" Jo emphasized.

"No, ma'am," he said. "She never lost her pulse."

To keep Lisa alive, Shocktrauma technicians hooked her to

a ventilator to pump oxygen into her lungs. Her body continued to survive.

At 11 P.M., nearly three hours after her accident, Lisa was transferred to Neurotrauma on the fourth floor, the ward for head and spinal-cord injuries. Martha Kowalski, the floor nurse who would care for her, came on duty as Lisa's stretcher was wheeled into Neurotrauma. A beautiful, broken bird, Martha thought as the stretcher rolled past. An arterial line inserted into Lisa's left arm gave a continuous readout of blood pressure and heartbeat on a digital monitor at the head of her bed. Both of these vital signs remained stable. A small computer at the nurses' station showed Lisa's blood gases, electrolyte levels, blood counts, and other lab values. Most were in the normal range.

Lisa's neurological status was checked again by a neurosurgeon. He tested her response to deep pain. She had none. He shined a thin beam of light into the retina of Lisa's right eye. This sent a message to the brain, which should send a return message to shut out the invading light, but Lisa's pupils remained fixed and dilated. Other tests sought to elicit other nerve and reflex responses, but they too failed to find any. Lisa was then taken off the ventilator momentarily to see if she could breathe spontaneously. This is perhaps the most basic of all human survival functions, and Lisa could not do it. Her brain had deteriorated markedly since admission.

Different states have different standards to measure brain death. In Maryland, where there is no requirement for electroencephalograph readings, these tests are how the determination of brain death is made. After he'd completed them, the neurosurgeon had no question that Lisa's brain was dead, and there was no hope of recovery.

Martha remained in Lisa's room and Jo appeared.

"How's she doing?" Jo asked.

"Stable," Martha answered. "Have you talked to her family?"

"Not yet," Jo said. "I'm just about to."

The floor was quiet. Martha watched the digital monitor and saw Lisa's blood pressure drop sharply, from 110 to 70, then down to 50. She injected Lisa with dopamine and pushed in more intravenous fluids to stabilize her blood pressure. Lisa was being kept alive for her organs.

Hospitals are always gloomy. Now, close to midnight, the empty halls smelling of stale antiseptic, this one seemed very cold and bleak. In the small waiting room outside Neurotrauma, Jo met Maureen, still wearing a parka and sitting alone on an old brown sofa. Her hands were folded in her lap. Maureen stood as Jo approached. Jo looked directly into her eyes; they were rimmed in red, but she was no longer crying. Maureen had an open, accepting face, Jo thought.

Jo introduced herself. "First I must tell you how very sorry I am," she said as she extended her hand to Maureen.

Maureen took her hand and thanked Jo for her sympathy. She explained to Jo that she was a nurse, and then said, "I'd like to see Lisa. I want to see if she looks well enough for my father to see her. I'm worried about him if she looks too bad." She gave Jo no sign that she harbored any hope for Lisa.

"I'll take you to her," Jo said, and led her to a supply room, where she helped her on with a sterile gown. Then she ushered her to Lisa's bedside. As soon as Maureen walked into the room and saw her little sister, she cried again. She leaned over the low railing and touched her and felt the coldness of her body. Lisa's temperature had dropped to 95 degrees. Martha walked over to Maureen's side and put her arm around her, and the three women watched silently.

They stepped outside Lisa's room, and Jo spoke to Maureen. "I wish I could tell you there was hope, but there isn't," she said. "I know the neurosurgeon has already told you that."

Maureen nodded.

"I'd like you to consider donating Lisa's organs," Jo said. "I

19

want you to do it, but I want you to do it for yourselves. As time passes, it will mean something to you that may help you deal with Lisa's loss."

Maureen appeared thoughtful as Jo spoke, but her instinct was to shout, "No! Don't hurt her any more!"

She calmly turned to Jo. "I'll have to ask Dad. He'll make the decision," she said.

Then she startled Jo. "Lisa is not my blood sister," she said. She explained that Lisa was a foster child who had always used the Kelly name and who, after a long legal struggle, was about to be adopted by the family.

"The adoption was supposed to be final next week," Maureen said quietly.

Jo did not betray her concern, and Maureen headed downstairs to the waiting room to find her father.

Donald Kelly, the oldest of the Kelly children, finally arrived at Shocktrauma. He had moved that day and his new phone had not been installed. When his wife's mother had finally reached him, he left immediately for the hospital.

Donald and Lisa had enjoyed a close relationship when they were younger. When Lisa was ordered to bed at night, she'd sneak into Don's room and stay up late watching television. He made up stories about himself for her, once convincing her that he wrote "Stop, In the Name of Love," a popular song by the Supremes. Every time the song played on the radio Lisa shouted, "That's Donny's song." He'd teased her about it for years.

Now as he ran down the corridor toward the waiting room, he was met by his mother, who was weeping.

"How's Lisa?" he asked.

"There's no hope," his mother told him. "She's gone."

"Oh, God," he shouted, and slammed his fist into the wall. Then his head dropped, and he turned and ran out of the hospital, not to return, not to mention her name for months.

When Maureen came back, she found her father waiting

quietly with her mother and Tom. He wanted to see Lisa one final time, he said, but he and Maureen agreed that Louise was not up to it. Maureen was worried about what seeing Lisa might do to her father, but he insisted, so Maureen led him toward the fourth floor. "You'd better stay with Mom," Maureen said to Tom as they left.

In organ donorship the permission of the next of kin is absolutely essential. This made Lisa's case complicated. The Kellys were Lisa's family, but the state was her legal guardian. Could the Kellys legally give permission to donate? Jo telephoned the state attorney general's office and finally reached a lawyer at home. He said the county director of human services was the one person who had the final say on organ donatio.

Jo called the director and woke him up. He was shocked and saddened to hear of the accident. He knew Lisa and her sister, he told Jo. He had just seen them last week. He agreed organ donation was appropriate but didn't want to overrule the family.

"If they agree to the donation, so will I," he told Jo. "They've been Lisa's real family for the past fourteen years."

"I wouldn't go against the family's wishes either, even if we could," Jo assured him. She hung up and headed back to Neurotrauma.

What first struck Jo when she saw Eugene Kelly coming down the corridor toward her was how much he resembled her own father; it was startling and unsettling. He was short and stocky, and he maintained a serenity and dignity in this terrible time.

"Mr. Kelly," Jo said as she approached him, "I'm so terribly sorry about this."

He nodded and thanked her. She helped him on with a sterile gown and led him to Lisa. He stood over her as she lay motionless, the ventilator breathing for her, thick bandages over her head and the side of her face.

Tears welled up in his eyes. Maureen wept again, and for

maybe a minute no one said a word. Only the hissing and pumping of the ventilator were audible.

"She was so alive," Maureen said, sobbing. "And so loving."

"She was our precious angel," Eugene Kelly said. His voice began to break. Martha Kowalski had seen many families in this situation. She'd seen them scream, faint, even deny the death. As she watched Maureen and her father, she saw how pained they were, but also how strong they were.

A few minutes later a Catholic priest arrived and gave Lisa the final sacrament of the sick. The Kellys had not been regular churchgoers, but they wanted Lisa to have the last rites.

Now Maureen leaned over and gently kissed Lisa on the forehead and whispered goodbye. Her father could not bring himself to do that. He touched Lisa on the arm and turned away as they left her bedside for the last time.

It was clear to Jo that the Kellys understood brain death. Although Lisa was breathing and her heart was beating, she would never again be what she was. Jo asked Mr. Kelly if he would consider donating Lisa's organs.

He didn't hesitate for a moment. "Yes, I think that would be proper. Lisa loved people and she always wanted to give to them."

Maureen, surprised at the suddenness of her father's decision, knew he was right. She looked at him and nodded her assurance. Jo was relieved.

Jo asked if Lisa was suffering from any disease or disorder.

"No," Eugene said, "she's always been very healthy."

Jo handed him a University of Maryland Hospital organ-donation form. It certified that he was who he said he was, and that he permitted the "anatomical gift" from Lisa. He signed it.

Maureen had one request. "Please, under no circumstances let my mother in to see Lisa. I think it would be too much for her."

22

Jo agreed. Eugene and Maureen also felt Louise should not know that they had agreed to donate Lisa's organs. Not now anyway. "That just would be too much for her," Eugene said.

"I won't tell her, and I'll make sure no one else does," Jo promised.

Jo told them both that there was nothing more they could do at the hospital. Lisa would be monitored throughout the night, and an official declaration of death would be made in the morning.

"Why don't you go home and get some rest," she told them.

Maureen and her father agreed, and Jo walked them to the elevator. They faced another difficult task. Ellen, who had gone out earlier in the evening, was not yet aware of Lisa's fatal accident and would have to be told. They found Louise and Tom in the waiting area and began their journey home. It was 2 A.M., and it was very cold.

Jo's physical and emotional exhaustion gave way to duty. She had gone into medicine because she had wanted to contribute, but her work took her into the grimmest of circumstances. As a physician's assistant, she had often performed minor surgery as well as hands-on patient care. She missed that aspect of her former work, talking to patients, caring for them. But this was important, and she was good at it. She worked coolly and methodically, following a procedure she'd been through scores of times. She went to the coffee room and got another cup. Soon she forgot how tired she was.

The next critical phase of organ transplantation was tissue typing. Throughout the complicated process she always had to fight time, the constant enemy. She returned to the pathology laboratory and learned that Lisa's kidney function was excellent. A toxicology screening was negative: Lisa had no drugs or alcohol in her system. Hemoglobin and hematocrit, two important measurers of blood, were normal. Electrolyte levels seemed stable. Everything was alive except Lisa's brain.

Brain-dead patients are difficult even for medical professionals. Some nurses describe them as eerie and unnerving. Even some physicians cannot or do not understand the concept of brain death. Jo had a running encounter with one young physician at Shocktrauma who refused to accept it. He believed if the heart was beating, the patient was alive and must not be declared dead. Court battles had been fought over the issue — the Karen Ann Quinlan case the most notable — and only in the past few years had brain death become a legally accepted definition of death. More than half of the states have passed laws defining brain death and how it must be determined medically. In states without such laws, the determination of brain death is often a decision reached by the physician and the next of kin.

Jo did not have any misgivings about brain death. She'd seen it often and accepted it as the end. But that did not make what she did any easier.

It was now past 3 A.M. Jo braced herself against the cold as she walked out the double glass doors that led to the parking area behind Shocktrauma. It was very quiet. She climbed into her VW bus, cranked over the engine, and backed out of her parking stall. She could see puffs of breath against the glare of her headlights as she headed across town to the tissue-typing lab at The Johns Hopkins Hospital, which performed the service for the region. She carried a small vial of Lisa Kelly's blood, enough for the tissue typing. She'd already notified the tissue typer; Hopkins had one on call twenty-four hours a day.

There are distinct tissue types among people, just as there are distinct blood types, but tissue types are much more complicated. Tissue types are identified by specific proteins found in cells in the body. They can be obtained readily from white blood cells. These proteins, called antigens, are part of the complex mechanism that defines self and nonself for the body, and that helps fight disease.

The major human antigen system is called the HLA, which stands for human leukocyte antigen. Located on the sixth chromosome, it is considered to be the most complex genetic system yet found in humans. It is also the system that determines our individual tissue type. It is clear that the better matched the tissue between donor and recipient, the better the chance the transplanted organ has to succeed. It is equally clear that what is known about tissue typing is a small fragment of what there is to know.

Dave Kappus, a young man casually dressed in a lab coat, jeans, and running shoes, was accustomed to his pager going off at all hours of the night; it was an occupational hazard. A biology major at Ohio State, he had been a tissue typer at Johns Hopkins for four years, working in the eighth-floor laboratory of the Traylor Building. Jo gave him Lisa's blood sample. She told him it was type A.

After a series of intricate steps, Kappus put the tube of blood on the centrifuge one last time, where it spun, leaving the heavier red cells at the bottom and a whitish layer of pure lymphocytes at the top. He sucked the lymphocytes, which contained the antigens he was looking for, into a pipette and put them on plates. This was the final stage of tissue typing, but results were still hours away.

Realizing she had a long day in front of her, Jo didn't stay for the entire tissue-typing process. "Call me," she said, leaving.

Kappus, alone in the lab, worked through the night.

Thirty miles away, in the stillness of their home, memories, questions, and pain kept Eugene and Louise Kelly awake. Eugene paced the floor for a while and then sat alone in a chair in the living room. At 4 A.M. he called Shocktrauma. He reached Martha Kowalski, who was still on duty.

"Has Lisa died yet?" he asked.

"No," Martha told him. "Lisa's status is unchanged."

He thanked Martha, hung up, turned to Louise, and told her there was no change.

"Then why are they keeping Lisa alive on the ventilator if there's no hope?" she asked.

He paused, looked at her with an expression she couldn't interpret, and shrugged. Now was not the time to tell her.

26

Jo unlocked her front door and went in. Rick had left a small kitchen light on. She hung up her coat, took off her shoes, and walked upstairs to the bedroom. Rick was sound asleep. She set her alarm for 7 A.M., slipped into her nightgown, and moved quietly into bed. Rick stirred and draped his arm around her and she nestled next to him.

She lay there, going over the still unfinished details of Lisa's case. She thought about the Kellys. Although she'd been in organ procurement for more than three years, recently she'd noticed a change in herself. At first she'd entered the field to help the recipients, those people out along the organ network who wait, often desperately, for a kidney, a liver, a heart, or a cornea. Some die waiting; some come close to nervous breakdowns. But now she realized she was really in it for the donor families. It was they she came to know and care about. And it was to them that she tried to bring fragments of meaning amid the randomness of sudden death.

Her work often tore at her emotions, putting hope and despair in precarious balance. She sensed the Kellys' pain, as she'd sensed the pain of many families. But she did not, or could not, acknowledge that pain in herself. If she let it all in, it could take over her life. She had to keep it in a separate place, out of reach. Above all else, she considered herself a professional.

She tried to sleep, but it didn't come easily.

The sky was turning light by the time Dave Kappus began to identify Lisa's tissue type. By a process of elimination, he identified three antigens, numbers one and three on what is called the A locus, and number seven on her B locus. The two loci identify the specific sites where the antigens are located on the chromosomes. Although four antigens are normally found at these two loci, Lisa apparently inherited an identical antigen from each parent, so only a total of three could be identified.

It was enough for proper tissue typing. Kappus entered his findings on the tissue-typing form.

In an IBM Series I computer in Richmond, Virginia, the headquarters of the Southeastern Region Organ Procurement Foundation, were the names of more than five thousand people from across the country. They were all waiting for an organ transplant. It was part of the United Network for Organ Sharing (UNOS), a computerized linkup of the country's more than one hundred and forty organ transplant centers. All these centers try to make the best possible use out of the relatively few human organs that become available for transplantation.

The list of five thousand represented only a portion of the people who needed a transplant. Many potential recipients were not listed on this particular day because they may have been too ill for a transplant operation; others voluntarily asked that their names be removed for a period of time for personal reasons; and transplant centers sometimes removed names for any number of reasons.

The list was updated daily. Some people on it were waiting for a heart or liver or a pancreas, but mostly it was made up of potential kidney recipients. Because kidney patients can be kept alive on dialysis while they wait, there were more of them. Some were waiting for their first transplant, some for their second or third. No matter the problems that may accompany an organ transplant, or the crushing disappointment of rejecting and losing one, kidney patients almost always are willing to gamble again for the chance at a more normal life. So they wait. It is their last, best hope.

Just before 8 A.M., in the corner of the Hopkins tissue-typing lab, Dave Kappus began typing in information about Lisa Kelly on the small terminal keyboard that feeds into UNOS. Age: 17; Race: White; Blood Type: A; and her tissue type.

The computer digested the information in seconds and then automatically gave back names, all in blood type A, in order

28

of priority. First was the "urgent" list on which thirteen names appeared. Eleven needed kidneys, one man in New York City needed a heart, another in Minneapolis needed a pancreas.

The country's major heart transplant center is at Stanford University. Because hearts can survive only a few hours outside the body, that was too far away to send one, even if there were a match. Livers and pancreases also won't last more than a few hours and are not transplanted nearly as often as kidneys. Many times they are obtained in the cities where the major liver and pancreas transplant centers are located, Pittsburgh and Minneapolis. But patients in need of a pancreas or liver often don't live very long, so the waiting lists are perishable. On the computer today, none of the people seeking a heart, liver, or pancreas matched tissues with Lisa.

Kappus scanned the names and looked for kidney matches on the urgent list. Only two had the minimum of a one-antigen match. As much as any single factor, the tissue and blood matching determine where a human organ will go. There is no point in sending a kidney or liver to a desperately ill patient if there is no match. The odds of rejection are too high.

After the urgent list, the computer ran through a second priority. It sought out perfect, four-antigen matches for anyone in the country in need of a kidney. However, because Lisa had only three identifiable antigens, the computer could not find any.

The next priority was local patients. The computer printed out the names of patients in the Baltimore area who needed a kidney. The names were arranged in order of their time on the waiting list and by the number of each patient's antigens that matched with Lisa's.

There were six possibilities. Kappus began cross-matching tests on all of the potential recipients. This was a final check on donor-recipient tissue compatibility done by mixing the white blood cells taken from Lisa with small blood samples of the waiting recipients that are kept at the Hopkins lab. He also had blood samples for other potential kidney recipients in the South-eastern Region, which covers transplant centers in fourteen states. In addition, he would do a limited number of cross-matches on potential cornea recipients.

At 8:15 A.M., across the city, a team of Shocktrauma physicians visited Lisa one final time. It was mandatory that they be separate and uninvolved with the transplant team so that a desire to find organs for transplant would not figure into their conclusions. They performed the same series of neurological tests they had performed the night before. Again there was no response, not a flicker of life. At 8:50 A.M., they pronounced Lisa Kelly dead of irreversible brain damage. It was a little more than twelve hours since her accident. She was kept on the ventilator, and intravenous fluids and drugs continued to stabilize her blood pressure and maintain her kidneys.

The tissue cross-matches of potential Baltimore kidney recipients showed none would succeed. The blue-stained cells Kappus saw in the tray wells meant the antigens Lisa carried in her white blood cells would stimulate the antibodies of the recipients; their bodies would probably reject her kidney immediately.

There were other possibilities in the Southeastern Region, and Kappus methodically performed the cross-matching tests on those potential kidney recipients for whom he had blood samples. One by one they were eliminated, but occasionally he found a waiting recipient that either had a good cross-match or for whom he had no blood sample and therefore didn't know if it would be a good or bad cross-match. When he finished later that morning, he called the hospital to have them get in touch with Jo. He would send over the computer printout he had marked for her.

Exhausted by two nearly sleepless nights, Jo overslept Sunday morning when her alarm failed to go off. At 9 A.M. her pager sounded. She phoned Shocktrauma and learned the printout was ready. The Kelly family also had been calling. "Come here as soon as you can," a harried nurse said.

"I'm on my way," Jo told her.

Rick stirred. "You have to go?"

"Afraid so," Jo said. "I can't believe I slept till nine."

Rick went downstairs and put on the coffee while Jo dressed. She gulped down a cup, kissed Rick goodbye, promised a quiet night at home, and was out the door. The Sunday morning sky was the color of lead and a light rain fell. She arrived at Shocktrauma at 9:30 and phoned Maureen, who told Jo that the family had just been told that Lisa had been officially declared dead.

"Should we come to the hospital?" Maureen asked.

"There's nothing for you to do here," Jo said. "You should tell the funeral director you've chosen that Lisa's body will be available later today, certainly by midafternoon."

"Have they taken out her organs yet?" Maureen asked.

"Not yet," Jo answered. "That will happen soon. I want to thank you again for your generosity, and for thinking of others at what I know is a terrible time for you. I also want to tell you again how sorry I am."

Maureen thanked Jo, and Jo realized Maureen had begun to cry again.

At 10:30 A.M., an hour and a half after the official declaration of death, Jo had found a surgeon, and secured permission to use an operating room. Lisa Kelly's body was wheeled into OR Six at the University of Maryland Hospital. All life-support systems continued. A young vascular-surgical resident made a long incision and began removing her kidneys. He was careful to leave the severed vessels and ureter long enough so that the

31

surgeons on the other end of the transplant procedure would be able to stitch them into the recipients easily.

Jo carefully placed Lisa's kidneys in two sterile plastic bags and put them in a styrofoam chest filled with chipped ice. She left the operating room and took an elevator to her sixth-floor office and laboratory. The temperature in the chest was kept at 4 degrees centigrade, about the temperature of a home refrigerator. Now that Lisa's kidneys were out of her body, time became more critical.

Jo went to the phone and called Bob Grant, another organ-procurement coordinator with her office. He had just arrived home after taking his family to church.

"How soon can you get here?" she asked. "We've got two kidneys to place."

"I'll be there in twenty minutes," he said.

With the tissue-typing printout provided by Dave Kappus, Jo and Bob began calling centers where patients had good matches with Lisa. It was already fifteen hours after Lisa's accident. Because Lisa was so young, Jo did not expect problems in placing the kidneys. One of the most promising matches was at the Vanderbilt Medical Center in Nashville, Tennessee. Jo phoned. She learned the patient at Vanderbilt was too ill for a transplant right now. Jo and Bob kept calling.

Recipients, when finally identified, are notified in all kinds of ways. Once a good match was found for a trucker. The problem was, he was on a long-haul run. Through state police, he was eventually pulled over several hundred miles from the transplant center, put in a private plane, and flown home. Another time, television stations cooperated by displaying the name of a potential recipient on the television screen until his family, together for a holiday, saw it and sent him off to the hospital. And then there was the young man from Waltham, Massachusetts, who was tracked down at the giant Live Aid concert in Philadelphia and flown back to Boston, where a kidney had just become available for him.

The list of potential recipients narrowed down to a three-year-old boy in Cincinnati. It was a three-antigen match, considered very good.

Jo called Ron Dreffer, the organ-procurement coordinator in Cincinnati. "I know of the family," he said. "They've had a lot of problems and they're very anxious for a kidney for their little boy. I'll get right back to you."

After checking with the doctor, Dreffer called Jo back. "We want the kidney," he said. "We really need it."

"You got it," Jo said. To accept it meant Cincinnati would pick up the five-thousand-dollar kidney-procurement bill. The cross-matches, the final test to see if the donor and recipient were compatible, would be done in Cincinnati.

Because the human body can function well on one kidney, Jo had one more available. There was a potentially good match at Walter Reed Army Medical Center in Washington, D.C., and when Bob Grant called there he learned they too wanted the kidney, for a patient just about to be placed on the computer's urgent list.

"If there's a good cross-match we'd want it for her," said Dan Smith, the Walter Reed organ-procurement coordinator. "She's having a lot of problems on dialysis."

She was the wife of an army officer. "If she can't use it," Smith said, "we'll take responsibility for placing it at another hospital."

Lisa Kelly's kidneys had both found homes.

The Medical Eye Bank is located in a three-story building with an awning on Park Street in downtown Baltimore. It is a private, nonprofit institution and the national leader in eye banking. It procures between four and five thousand eyes a year for cornea transplantation as well as research and medical training.

It was early Sunday afternoon when Bernard Madison, a medical technician there, received a call. There was a donor at the University of Maryland Hospital. He picked up his equipment and drove there in ten minutes.

Unlike kidneys, for which the body must still be alive when they are removed for transplantation, corneas can be procured up to twelve hours after death. Madison, a graduate in zoology from Howard University in Washington, D.C., approached Lisa in the operating room. Her kidneys removed, and all life-support systems turned off, she was no longer alive in any way.

A tall, quiet man, Madison performed his task with practiced precision. Like the kidneys, the corneas needed to be transplanted quickly, no more than forty-eight hours from the moment he removed them. Back at the Medical Eye Bank laboratory, Madison examined the corneas under a high-intensity slit lamp. They were in excellent condition — no cloudiness, no damage of any kind. He treated both corneas with an antibiotic and phoned the office of Dr. Walter Stark, an ophthalmologist and cornea-transplant surgeon at Johns Hopkins.

Dr. Stark was involved in a national research project in which corneas were matched between donor and recipient, the same way kidneys were. This had not been done regularly because corneas normally have no blood supply, and thus it was thought they were "privileged," that is, they would not be rejected as a result of antibodies carried in the bloodstream. But corneas do get rejected, especially in people who have already rejected one cornea transplant. So Stark wanted to find out if tissue matching would improve their functioning and survival.

Corneas are shared between cornea-transplant specialists in much the way kidneys are, but the sharing system is less formal. The Eye Bank did not have a computerized system, only a written list of potential recipients.

Madison reached a nurse with Dr. Stark's office. She examined a list of potential recipients who were waiting for a tissue-matched cornea transplant. She had in front of her the cross-match tests performed by Dave Kappus at the tissue-typing lab.

"There are no good matches in our area," she told Madison.

She also had the names of patients at the Massachusetts Eye and Ear Infirmary, which was participating in the tissue-matching study. Two patients there appeared to cross-match well. She called Boston and then called Madison back.

"Boston wants them both," she said.

Jo continued her race against time. On the side of the cooler that was to carry Lisa's right kidney on the hour-long car trip to Walter Reed Army Medical Center was a bright orange sign with bold black lettering that read: HUMAN KIDNEY FOR TRANSPLANT. For the longer trip to Cincinnati Children's Hospital — and because the physicians there demanded it — Jo placed Lisa's left kidney on a perfusion machine in which a cooled mixture of plasma, saline solution, dextrose, and other nutrients was pumped through the vessels of the kidney to simulate normal circulation. Jo was allergic to the perfusion fluid and she always had red blotches on her hands and wrists from it.

There were potential problems that worried her. She was not certain of the cross-match with either of the kidney recipients. If one or both of them didn't work out, the kidneys might have to be sent to other centers — more time lost. And there was always the possibility that the kidneys would be out of the body too long to be used.

Jo very much wanted the kidneys to be used, to sustain life in other people. These people would only be names to her; people who, because of an act of kindness by a bereaved family, would have a chance at a normal life. And she wanted the kidneys placed because she hoped one day their use would help the Kellys deal with Lisa's loss.

She called the airlines. "Do you have any flights to Cincinnati this afternoon?"

The answer was no more commercial flights between Baltimore and Cincinnati today.

She called a charter service. "Can you get me a charter to Cincinnati this afternoon?"

They could, and she booked a twin-engine Navaho.

The organ-procurement people in the recipient cities prepared to rendezvous at the airports to pick up the incoming kidneys and corneas. They were as conscious of time as Jo.

Sunday afternoon in their living room, a room dominated by a large fieldstone fireplace and pictures of their family, the Kellys talked quietly. The high school picture on the mantel of Lisa was next to one of her sister Ellen. Ellen had worn a stunned expression throughout the day and had said little. Several times she'd asked why Lisa had been walking along that stretch of road; it was the only question she seemed able to ask right now. The Kellys all took special care with her, realizing how devastating Lisa's loss was for her.

Friends and neighbors had come by the Kelly home to offer condolences. Maureen stayed all day to help her parents through it.

An acquaintance of Louise Kelly came by and stayed for several minutes. A pleasant woman, just about Louise's age, she talked of the loss of her son several years earlier to kidney disease.

"He wouldn't have lived even that long except for the kidney someone donated to him," she said. "It gave him a few extra years, and we were grateful for that."

Eugene Kelly listened to the conversation and sensed the time was now right. He approached his wife, put his arm around her, and told her that he'd already given permission to donate Lisa's organs.

"I didn't tell you before because I was afraid it would upset you," he told her.

Louise looked at her husband. She now understood why Lisa had been kept on the ventilator all night at Shocktrauma. She put her hand to his face and spoke softly: "It doesn't upset me. I had thought about it too, but I didn't say anything because I thought it would upset you."

~~~~~~~~~~~~~~~~ T H R E E

I t was a quiet Sunday afternoon. The sun was bright and a
hard wind was pushing cold air through Ohio and much
of the Midwest. Scattered over the landscape were small, icy
crusts of snow, the remains of a late February storm. Despite
the cold, Jim Landis worked up a heavy sweat splitting wood
in his backyard. He was a stocky, square-shouldered man in his
early thirties, of medium height, with a round, friendly face.
He drove his newly sharpened ax into the hickory and oak logs
with power and precision. He was exceptionally skilled with his
hands and worked as a millwright at a nearby cosmetics plant,
where he repaired the production machines.

Every autumn he went into the woodlands of nearby Indiana
with his younger brother Carl and two chain saws and hauled
back a truckload of logs for his wood stove. By choice, this stove
was the only source of home heating during the cold Ohio
winters. "Sometimes the house even gets too warm," he was
fond of saying. "You can't control it with a thermostat, so there
are days in the dead of winter we have to open the windows to
cool the place down."

His home was a three-bedroom split-level in a new residential
suburb outside Cincinnati. The land rolled gently and there
was plenty of open space. It was a good area for young families.

Jim and his wife, Betty, had worked hard for the house. Jim
had put in hours of overtime until they'd saved enough for the

down payment. He'd remodeled one room, nurtured the lawn, and fixed everything that broke. He and Betty took pride in their home and in their family of three children.

Jim carried an armload of wood from his backyard to a place near the stove and heard the telephone ring.

"I'll get it," Betty shouted.

She recognized the caller immediately: it was Dr. Paul McEnery from Cincinnati Children's Hospital. "Could you bring Matthew down here this afternoon?" he asked. "We'd like to draw some blood for a cross-match. We've got a kidney coming in from Baltimore, and it looks pretty good."

Betty cupped her hand over the phone and called to Jim, "It's Dr. McEnery; they've got a kidney coming." Jim felt a surge of excitement and nodded to Betty.

"We'll be down there as fast as we can," Betty said. "Give us an hour."

"I'll be here," McEnery told her.

They made hasty arrangements with Jim's mother to watch Valerie and Janie, their two daughters. Matthew, their youngest child, was in his room, contentedly playing with blocks. Posters of Batman, Wonder Woman, and Superman were on the walls, and around the room were a variety of stuffed animals. Sitting on his bed, next to his pillow, was his special stuffed animal, the monkey Curious George. Betty knelt down next to Matthew.

"Matthew, Dr. McEnery just called."

Matthew took no notice, although he knew who Dr. McEnery was.

"He wants us to come to the hospital, just for a test. It won't take very long."

Matthew turned to her. He could read her face and Betty knew it, so it was always fruitless to lie, or even to soft-pedal anything to him.

"A stick?" he asked.

Betty knew Matthew hated and feared sticks, his word for

needles. He'd even had nightmares about them. "Yes, honey," she told him, "but just a little one, and Mommy and Daddy will be there."

"We go now?" he said, without changing expression.

"Yes, we have to go now."

"I get George," he said.

"Oh, yes," Betty said, "I think George wants to come too."

Matthew reached over and grabbed Curious George by the arm. He always wanted him when he went to the hospital or needed comforting. He'd spent nearly a quarter of his young life in the hospital, and he always accepted going there with an outward calm. He seemed to understand that sometimes he needed to be there.

Although five months away from his fourth birthday, Matthew was closer in size to a two-year-old because his congenital kidney problem had slowed his growth. He had brown hair with a tinge of red, and his small torso showed the scars of several operations. He'd already had two failed kidney transplants, and both of those kidneys had been removed. One rejection was so severe it brought him to the brink of death. His face was round, almost cherubic, and his eyes were a deep, rich brown. They seemed to absorb everything and held a sad wisdom beyond their years.

Most adults awaiting a kidney transplant survive on kidney dialysis. Matthew was different. Unlike an adult, he could not be saved with dialysis because his blood vessels were too small to tolerate it for all but the shortest time. Even if they could, he would never grow on dialysis. He needed a successful kidney transplant to live, and thrive. Because he'd rejected two, it was very possible that the third one would be his final chance.

Matthew was only alive because a very small part of the one natural kidney he was born with still functioned. But that kidney, which was congenitally defective, was failing. No one had predicted how long it would last, or how long Matthew would live, but his time was running out.

Jim and Betty knew all this and had lived with it for a long time. As hard as it was at times, they'd never given up hope.

They packed all three children in Jim's Dodge Challenger, a car he'd rebuilt himself, and headed toward Jim's parents' home, a short drive away. His mother, Edna Landis, walked out of her house and greeted Valerie, who was nine, and Janie, six, as they ran toward her.

She approached the car and peeked in at Matthew. "Hi there, honeybunch."

Matthew turned to her and smiled, then rolled his head toward Betty, who held him in her lap.

Edna spoke to Jim. "They can stay the night if that'll help."

"Thanks, but I expect this won't take too long. But if it goes like I hope it will, we'll be calling you a lot in the next few days."

Edna Landis squeezed Jim's arm. "You know I'm always here."

Jim smiled. Betty thanked Edna, and they backed out of the driveway. Sunday traffic was light. They'd made the half-hour trip from their home to Children's countless times. Some had been worried trips, others dire emergencies; this one was hopeful.

Matthew sat comfortably in his mother's lap. "You feeling okay, honey?" she asked him.

"Yeah," he answered in a soft voice. She squeezed him in her arms and kissed him lightly atop his head. He looked at the passing landscape and remained quiet.

Jim glanced over at Matthew and smiled, then reached over to touch him. "We're gonna be with you all the time, Matthew," Jim said. Matthew just looked at him.

Although his life was a restricted one, in every important way

Matthew was a normal three-year-old. He loved to visit his grandparents, play in the dirt, be his daddy's helper, and watch cartoons on television. He especially loved to paint, and his artwork was pasted all over the kitchen refrigerator.

Betty clutched Matthew as the car moved along a narrow road on the way to the interstate and downtown Cincinnati. Betty was shyer and more intense than Jim. At one time she wanted to work in medicine, but after her marriage and the birth of Valerie, she devoted herself to caring for her family.

She had an intelligent face, dark-rimmed glasses, and soft brown eyes. She and Jim had grown up right next door to one another, only a few blocks from where they now lived. Betty was an adopted, only child, and Jim was a member of a large family. Betty had never especially liked Jim when they were young, but after he returned from his navy hitch an attraction developed. They dated for a while and in 1969 they were married. He was twenty and she was eighteen, just out of high school.

Both wanted a family and they enjoyed their children. They regularly took them on trips, out fishing, to church and Sunday school, and to Sunday afternoon barbecues at the children's grandparents. And during summer when the kids had no school and Jim worked the second shift and seldom saw them, he often went into their bedrooms after work at 2 A.M. and gently spoke to them, to let them know that he was there.

Jim stopped for a red light and looked over at Matthew. "How's my little man?" he asked, touching his son's tiny hand. Matthew smiled weakly.

"Just one stick?" Matthew asked.

"Yes, Matthew," Betty assured him, "just one stick. No more."

Matthew seemed content with that answer. He lay his head against Betty's shoulder and she hummed the alphabet song to him. He was always comforted by her soft singing voice.

Both Jim and Betty's most optimistic emotions had been tempered by the three-year struggle they and Matthew had endured. Betty had reached the point where she now fought against hoping too much, because it only invited deeper disappointment.

Just three weeks earlier, Cincinnati Children's Hospital, one of the national leaders in pediatric kidney transplants, had called with an ideally matched kidney for Matthew. Jim and Betty rushed him down only to find that he had a urinary tract infection, common in kidney patients. Because the drugs needed for the transplant suppressed his immune system, the infection could run rampant. Twenty minutes before surgery his transplant operation was canceled. That was only the most recent disappointment.

All had appeared normal at Matthew's birth. He seemed a robust, healthy baby and he thrived for the two months Betty was able to breast-feed him. He was built along the same sturdy lines as his father.

At three months, there was a change that was so gradual only Betty's intuition picked it up at first. Matthew didn't want to be held, and he began to spit up formula. When she switched to another type, he spit that up too. He ran an occasional fever, then it would mysteriously disappear. Visits to the pediatrician were inconclusive. He told Betty that Matthew probably had a virus. This vague array of symptoms persisted. Then Betty and Jim worried because Matthew was not growing normally. The pediatrician said Matthew would be a small person and told Betty not to worry.

At the age of five-and-a-half months Matthew came down with bronchitis. Not easily alarmed, Betty became frightened as his fever rose to 104 degrees. She visited another pediatrician, who wanted Matthew examined at Children's Hospital, immediately. Fear crept into Jim and Betty's thoughts, but it was outweighed by the belief that once Matthew's problem was diagnosed, it could be cured.

At 6:30 A.M. on a Saturday in November, the morning after

Matthew's admission to Children's Hospital, their new pediatrician called. He said specialists had completed their examination of Matthew.

"What did you come up with?" Jim asked.

Jim could hear the pause in the doctor's voice. "Matthew was born with only one kidney and it's badly diseased. I'm afraid he's close to total kidney failure."

When Jim hung up the phone he turned to Betty to tell her what he'd just learned, but he couldn't finish a sentence.

During Matthew's fetal development, two kidneys apparently had formed into one large, abnormal kidney, and the ureter, the tube that drains urine from the kidney into the bladder, was double its normal length and had looped and knotted. This caused urine to back up into his kidney. Matthew's first operation removed the knot and maintained the small kidney function he had left, at least for a while. His kidney's filtering system had also become clogged with cow's milk from his formula, and that meant Matthew needed a special diet.

Although Jim and Betty thought if they — or their original pediatrician — had acted sooner Matthew might have been spared some of his kidney problems, none of the doctors supported this idea. Even if Matthew had been properly diagnosed the day of his birth, nothing could have helped his one defective kidney.

Jim now drove down Bethesda Avenue toward the entrance of Children's Hospital, with its long, blue awning. He parked the car and lifted Matthew into his arms, and they took an elevator to the kidney unit on Three South. Dr. McEnery, a tall, friendly man in his midforties, greeted them.

"Hi there, Matthew," he said. "How you doing?"

"Okay," Matthew said shyly.

"We've got to take a little blood, Matthew," McEnery said. "I know you don't like that but we have to do it. Okay?"

Matthew nodded affirmatively.

44

Only one favored nurse, Monica Quinlan, could take Matthew's blood without causing him to cry. She was not on duty this Sunday afternoon.

A young nurse approached Matthew as he sat on an examining table with Betty holding one of his hands and Jim encouraging him to be brave. "This will just be a little stick, Matthew. I'll try not to hurt too much, okay?"

Matthew nodded, but still did not speak.

"Which arm do you want me to do it with?" she asked.

He held out his left arm and gave her a suspicious look. She rolled back his sleeve, swabbed a small area, and gingerly slid in the needle. Matthew hugged Curious George extra hard and fought back tears. It was over quickly. A small vial of his blood was taken immediately to the lab.

Jim, who had taught himself much about kidney transplants, asked McEnery about the tissue match.

"It's a three-antigen match," McEnery told him, "and we've been told it's a small kidney, which is good news indeed. We should be able to fit it into Matthew with no problem."

Jim asked about the donor, and McEnery told him the age, sex, and area where she was from. In organ transplantation, the names of the donor family and the recipient are not revealed to one another. Confidentiality is one reason. So is the fear that the donor family could grieve twice if they got to know the recipient, and the recipient either rejected the organ or died.

"When will you know about the cross-match?" Jim asked.

"We're still waiting for the kidney to get here, so it'll be a few hours. I'll call you. No sense for you to hang around here."

Matthew walked around the kidney unit, where he was something of a celebrity. He'd read everyone's expressions and knew this was not going to be a bad visit.

"Hi there, Matthew," a nurse called out. "Got George with you, I see."

Matthew smiled. "I had a stick."

She smiled, leaned down and patted him, said she was sorry, and walked away.

Matthew spoke in a babyish way, as do many young children who have had long hospital confinements during speech development. But he was understandable, and because so many of the staff realized he'd been through so much, and because he was so cute, he'd become a favorite.

Betty finished talking with Dr. McEnery and found Matthew at the nurses' station. He was watching the buttons on the telephone light up.

"You want to stay here and help the nurses, Matthew?" Betty asked.

Matthew remained preoccupied with the phones as Betty approached closer. "Time to go home now. You want to go home, don't you?"

"Yeah, we go home now," he answered.

Betty reached over and scooped him up in her arms and told him to say goodbye to everyone.

"Bye-bye," he said. Then he grabbed Curious George's arm and flapped it back and forth. "George say goodbye too," Matthew announced. Several nurses smiled and waved goodbye back to him.

The three of them left Children's to await McEnery's call. They'd spent a good part of their lives waiting for phone calls about Matthew.

A soft, silver glow on the western horizon was all that remained of the sunlight. Jim and Betty both felt the same sense of apprehension as they walked toward the parking lot. Matthew needed a kidney to live, and they were willing to expend every last effort for him. The transplantation of human organs was the medicine of last resort, but it was also the medicine of great possibilities.

Jim and Betty, braced against the cold, said little as they

walked. Their emotions had become so identical through the three-year ordeal that they were often unable to give each other much comfort.

"The caw," Matthew said, pointing to the red Challenger.

"You found the car, Matthew!" Jim shouted. "Great!"

Matthew smiled.

Once in the car, Matthew crawled into Betty's lap. "Now that wasn't too bad, was it?" she asked.

"Nope," he said, still holding Curious George. She wrapped her arms around him and held him close to keep him warm. He felt frail to her.

Jim drove along the streets leading from Children's. He remembered the time of Matthew's first kidney transplant two years earlier when, by chance, he and Betty met the parents of the little boy whose accidental death that same day gave Matthew a kidney.

They came upon one another in a hospital corridor, and when their eyes met they knew immediately who each other was. The little boy's mother moved toward them. "He's so beautiful," she said of Matthew, and reached out to touch him.

All in tears, they spoke briefly. "I'm so terribly sorry," Jim said, and he and Betty thanked them for their kindness and generosity in donating their son's kidney. "We wish you good luck," the little boy's father said, and then he and his wife left.

It was dark enough for headlights as Jim drove along the entrance ramp to the interstate. Matthew was curled in his mother's arms, sleepy but still awake. Jim knew the donor who might save his son's life was a seventeen-year-old girl killed in an accident near Baltimore. Our hope, he thought, is another family's pain.

At the front of the one-room church in Springfield, Massachusetts, was a cross made of two-by-fours, and near it was a large, red banner with the words MOVED BY HIS LOVE. The pews were simple, but it had taken the church a long time to raise the money for them. Throughout the service, already two hours old, the tiny congregation of two dozen men and women spontaneously cried out, "Thank You Jesus," "Amen," and "Praise the Lord." When the minister, a tall, forceful woman, led them in prayer, they prayed fervently, their eyes shut tight, clutching one another's hands. Other times they raised their arms, as if trying to touch the Holy Spirit they sensed moving among them. They sang to the simple beat of a tambourine or to a piano. Some fell to their knees and gave "testimony," a living witness to the power of God. The emotion and spirituality in the room was palpable at times.

Outside in the cold Massachusetts night, a man moved quickly toward the church. He could hear the joyful voices from inside. He walked to the front entrance and pounded on the door. The members were startled. The minister halted the service, then opened the door. She didn't recognize the man, who was lean and black. He stepped up and asked in a loud voice, "Is Derrick Jackson here?"

Derrick Jackson, sitting toward the rear of the church, heard but could not see. The voice was so commanding he thought for a second it must be the police. Why would the police want me now? he wondered.

"Is anything wrong?" the minister asked.

"No," the man said. "Nothing wrong."

As Derrick walked slowly toward the door, the voice became familiar. It was his older brother, David.

"Derrick," David said. "Boston called. They said they been trying to reach you all afternoon. Said they have a cornea for you."

Derrick almost jumped with excitement. He pulled on a heavy wool sweater and turned to Shirley Wright, who had been sitting next to him.

"Gotta go," he told her, touching her gently on the shoulder.

48

She read the eagerness in his face. "I'll pray for you," she said.

Shirley watched him walk away and smiled to herself. Derrick had put his sweater on backwards. She and Derrick had grown close over the past several months. They talked daily on the phone, he was very kind to her three young children, and she'd spent hours reading aloud to him from the Bible. She knew how badly he wanted to read the Bible himself. The congregation gathered in a circle around Derrick to wish him well and pray for him. Shirley moved forward to be with them, and as she did, a Biblical passage kept repeating in her mind: "If there is a knock on the door, it must be answered."

"Take my arm," David offered.

Derrick grabbed hold, feeling his way over the uneven terrain. Even in the best of light, he saw the world as if through waxed paper. The cause was congenital hereditary endothelia dystrophy, a disease that destroyed his corneas and made them appear as whitish, cloudy disks in the middle of his eye. The cornea covers the outer surface of the eye, much like a crystal covers a watch face.

Derrick could detect light and dark, and he saw large shapes, but never printed words, or faces, or details of any kind. He was legally blind; and he lived in fear of crossing the street at night.

About 5′9″ and reedy thin, he was twenty-three. He had never known his father. When he was young, his mother and her six children had moved to Springfield, an old manufacturing city in the western part of the state, where he grew up and still lived. For much of his life his world had been tightly circumscribed by bus routes and places to which he could walk. He was quiet, and although he often went for long periods of time without speaking a word, he was friendly and approachable.

Derrick knew what it was to see, even though his eyes had been damaged at birth. He'd received his first of four cornea transplants when he was five. Each of the transplanted corneas had worked for anywhere from a few months up to a year and a half, but each was eventually rejected, and his sight deteriorated. They had succeeded long enough for him to learn to read, and this had been his one pleasure in life. His most recent transplant was more than two years ago, but that had failed within a year. He was now unable to read anything.

While in special classes in elementary school, he'd hurled Braille learning cards across the room and wouldn't use them again. He would not use a Seeing Eye dog or a white cane. He refused to surrender to the idea that he wouldn't see again.

"You're a hard man to find," David said as they drove toward their mother's home.

"Spend all day Sunday at church," Derrick answered. "That's where you can usually find me."

They both realized that a few months earlier, Derrick was more likely to be found drunk than praying in a church. Derrick and his brother grew silent, and the only sounds were the humming of the car engine and the quick rushes of air as the car sped past the guardrail posts.

By his sophomore year in high school, Derrick was drinking alcohol and smoking marijuana regularly. His mother, as well as his sisters and brothers, tried to change him, but they could not reach him. There seemed to be a rage and a sense of isolation in him they could not penetrate. By his senior year in high school, Derrick was dealing drugs to other students, and after high school his life did not improve.

He worked fitfully at odd jobs when his sight permitted. He swept floors or packed boxes. But no job ever lasted for more than a few weeks. His mother, weary of him coming home drunk at all hours of the night, asked him to leave. He lived around the Springfield area, usually sharing apartments with other people. He snorted cocaine and heroin and used a variety of other drugs. He loved mescaline best because it removed him so completely from the world. When he and some friends were riding around once, they were stopped by police and a search revealed that there was a dangerous weapon in the car. Derrick said the gun wasn't his, and he didn't even know it was there, but he and the others were found guilty. On the day of his sentencing, the judge knew how poor Derrick's sight was and said he wouldn't last a week in prison. He gave Derrick three years' probation.

For the next few years, Derrick survived on his social security disability payment of $400 a month and spent much of it on beer, and most of his time drinking it. He also smoked cigarettes and marijuana regularly.

But on a hot, sultry afternoon the previous July, a day Derrick would never forget, his life changed. Unknown to him, Shirley Wright had watched Derrick from her kitchen window for months. She'd seen him sell beer to minors and drink himself into oblivion sitting on the front steps of her neighbor's house. Her neighbor's son was a friend of Derrick's. She'd also heard one neighborhood child taunt Derrick about his eyes.

She realized he was never abusive or violent, and she was troubled and touched by him. A few years earlier, she had been "saved" and had become a born-again Christian. She'd prayed for Derrick and was eager to share her faith with him. She felt a sense of mission about it. A tall, attractive woman in her late twenties, she had brown hair, an accepting face, and a direct look in her eyes. On that hot afternoon, she was moved to act. She asked her young daughter Elizabeth to go outside and invite Derrick into their home.

"My mother wants to see you," Elizabeth told Derrick.

He knew who Elizabeth was. She was the daughter of the woman who had never accepted a beer when he'd offered it to her.

"What'd you want to see me about?" he asked Shirley.

"You probably are going to think I'm crazy, but I've been

51

praying for you and the Lord wants me to tell you of His healing power."

Derrick could only make out the hazy outlines of her face. Maybe she is crazy, he thought. But he was curious. Why had she picked him out to tell all this mumbo-jumbo to?

"I know you're lonely," Shirley said.

Of course he was lonely, he thought. He'd always been lonely. He was a freak.

"I think the Lord passed me by," Derrick said, half smiling.

"He doesn't pass anyone by," Shirley answered.

She told him hard truths about himself, that he was close to alcoholism, if he wasn't already there; that his scrapes with the law, and his estrangement from his family, could not all be blamed on his failed sight.

"Your life doesn't have to be like this. There is a better way," she said.

Although his mind was clouded by alcohol, he felt some of the sting of what she said. She sounded so certain to him that despite the fact she was virtually a stranger, he didn't want to walk away.

They sat down in her living room and talked. Shirley read from the Bible and Derrick listened. Finally, she coaxed a promise out of him. He would attend church with her tomorrow.

"It's been a long time since I've been in church," he told her.

"I'll pick you up at six o'clock," she said.

That next night in the church, Derrick listened and observed as best he could. He felt moved by the strong sense of fellowship in the room, and the aura of a divine presence. The more he sat there, the more he felt that presence. He walked to the front of the church and felt overwhelmed by it. He slumped to the floor and wept. Derrick had been born again, that suddenly, that profoundly.

Right after that, he visited his mother, a quiet woman who taught nursery school. All her other children had become successful. One was a nurse, one an electronics technician, another a salesman; only Derrick seemed still to be drifting. He walked into his mother's living room and announced, "I've been saved."

She eyed him suspiciously. "Have you been drinking?"

"No, Mama, not a drop. The Lord is working in my life."

From that time on, Derrick never had a sip of alcohol, puff of a cigarette, or drug of any kind. He'd also made another commitment.

Several months before his religious conversion, just after his last cornea transplant had failed, he went to the Massachusetts Eye and Ear Infirmary, where he'd received his cornea transplants. A young doctor there examined him and then turned to Derrick and said, "As far as I'm concerned, you'll never get another cornea transplant."

"Why?" Derrick asked.

The doctor's voice was hard. "Because you don't take care of them, that's why. You miss your appointments, you don't put the drops in your eye, you act as if the transplant is some kind of lark for you. I'll tell you, there are a lot of other people who need a transplant just as much as you do, and they're willing to take care of themselves."

Derrick was angry and defensive. He stalked out of the examining room, muttering under his breath. But soon after his religious conversion, he took the bus back to Boston and met with the director of the Eye and Ear Infirmary. He explained his earlier encounter and admitted he had been negligent with his transplants in the past. But he was different now, he said. "If I'm ever lucky enough to get another cornea transplant," he said, "I'll treat it right. And I won't miss any appointments, either."

The director accepted Derrick's word. That day a nurse drew

a blood sample from Derrick, and he became part of Dr. Stark's tissue-matching study. He'd be called the moment they found an appropriate match, he was told.

David opened the car door and helped Derrick toward the entrance of their mother's home. Once inside, Derrick became exuberant. "I had a feeling something was gonna happen today. All things come to he who waits. I guess that's really true." He called the Eye and Ear Infirmary and told them he was on his way. His mother checked the bus schedule. The next one left at 9:15, an hour later.

Beth, the sister closest to Derrick, arrived. "Don't worry about the bus," she said. "I'll drive you."

He collected everything he needed and within minutes they were heading east on the Massachusetts Turnpike. The city lights of Springfield gave way to the rolling landscape of rural New England. "Bad thing about this," Derrick said, "is that someone had to die so I can get a cornea. But you can't question the Lord, I know he has a greater plan."

He fell silent in the front seat, praying for himself, and for the unknown donor and her family, whose gift might give him sight.

"Linda . . . it's me, Mom." Carolyn spoke in a whisper.

Linda's long blond hair languished on the pillow. She didn't move. Again Carolyn gently rocked her and whispered.

"I want to say goodbye, Linda. The hospital just called. They have the kidney for me. . . . Dad's driving me in. . . . He'll be back soon."

Linda nodded and reached up to embrace her mother.

"Take care of yourself, sweetheart, I'll call you from the hospital every day."

Linda cleared her throat and spoke. "What time is it?"

"It's almost midnight," Carolyn answered.

"I love you, Mom," Linda said.

"I love you too, very much," Carolyn said, with a parting hug.

Carolyn Blanchard, forty, a tall, trim woman with short brown hair and deep green eyes, tiptoed down the hall to Greg's room and flicked on his night-light. The room was outfitted with a stereo and headphones, and posters of rock stars hung on the walls. At sixteen, Greg was one year older than Linda. He woke up quickly when Carolyn touched him.

"I'm sorry to wake you, Greg, but I'm going to the hospital now."

Greg put his arms around Carolyn's neck and squeezed. He told her he'd worry about her, and she knew he would.

"When will you be back home?"

"It shouldn't be too long. I'm going to get out of there as soon as I can. Dad will be around to take care of things."

She hugged him, whispered, "I love you," and got up to leave. "I love you too," he called to her. She walked to the living room, where her husband, Tom, was waiting with his coat on. "I'm ready," she said.

Five years earlier, in Korea during one of Tom's tours of duty, Carolyn had stood on a long, winding stairway gasping for breath. Her home was at the top of the stairs, and she told herself she had to get up there, but her legs wouldn't move. She'd known it was coming. For weeks the climb had become harder, and she'd had throbbing headaches and nosebleeds. She'd known since her late teens that her kidneys were on borrowed time, and now time had run out. She leaned against the railing. The only sound she heard was the pounding of her heart.

She went to the local clinic. They told her that her blood pressure was 220 over 150 — dangerously high — and that she was in kidney failure. She was too ill to take care of Greg and Linda, and she needed the sophisticated treatment facilities available in the United States, so she had to leave them behind with their father and their live-in housekeeper. Within hours, arrangements were made for her to be airlifted to a U.S. hospital in her native California.

At the airport, so ill she could not stand up, she said goodbye to her children. Greg, then eleven, looked at her with frightened eyes and said, "Mom, I sure hope you'll make it."

"I'll make it," she told him, but as she labored to breathe, she wasn't certain she would.

She looked back at her children and Tom, as she was wheeled toward the waiting airplane, and felt a sense of loss she would never get over.

The kidney is the body's chemical regulator, controlling the electrolytes such as potassium. It also controls the fluid balance in the body, but its major function is to filter out the impurities that are natural by-products of our metabolism. These impurities are carried in the bloodstream and enter the kidney through the renal artery. Once inside the kidney, the blood traverses a series of little filtering cups called glomeruli. If the glomeruli from a pair of human kidneys were placed end to end, they would stretch fifty to sixty miles. It is within these glomeruli that waste products are separated from the blood and then excreted from the body in the form of urine.

When Carolyn was seventeen, she took a routine physical examination before going off to college at the University of California. The laboratory tests found she suffered glomerulonephritis. One of the more common of the serious kidney diseases, it caused the glomeruli in her kidneys to become inflamed. The process was like a long, smouldering infection, and over the years her kidney's filtering capacity was gradually destroyed. Carolyn had no symptoms at first because the kidney has an enormous reserve capacity, and most of us can survive with only 5 or 10 percent of our kidney function. But at the age of thirty-five, in Korea, Carolyn's kidneys had given out and could no longer perform even the most basic functions.

Her slow kidney disintegration had many costs, but none so painful as the two babies Carolyn brought to full term, only to lose at birth. Greg and Linda were both adopted.

In a Los Angeles hospital, Carolyn had remained on the critical list for two weeks after arriving there from Korea. What saved her life was hemodialysis, a process that filters blood mechanically. As miraculous as the hemodialysis device is, it punished Carolyn's heart and blood vessels because of the pressures it exerts on the body's vessels. It does this to all kidney patients who use it. Most hemodialysis patients die of heart failure. Also, because protein-breakdown products are cleared by the kidneys, Carolyn was restricted to the equivalent of only two ounces of meat a day. Fluid intake was also tightly restricted. Kidneys excrete potassium, a vital element in the transfer of electrical charges in the cells. Because potassium could not be regulated by her kidneys, she had to sharply reduce her intake of fruits, vegetables, orange juice, and other potassium-rich foods. She paid another price for hemodialysis: twice in the past year she'd suffered fluid overloads. Once, her lungs filled so quickly she was barely able to be resuscitated at an emergency room near her home.

Since Carolyn had moved to the Washington, D.C., area four years earlier — when Tom was transferred there after his Korean duty ended — she'd been seen by Dr. Jimmy Light, head of the Army-Navy transplant team at Walter Reed Army Medical Center in the northwest section of the city. Dr. Light had urged Carolyn to seek a kidney transplant ever since their first meeting, but she'd refused. She realized the longer she remained on dialysis, the more chancy the transplant's success would be, but for five years she had one unwavering answer: "I left my children once, and I've promised them, and myself, that I would never do that again until they were old enough to care for themselves." How could she forget the look in little Greg's eyes that day she boarded the plane in Korea?

In the past four months, she noticed short walks exhausted her. She'd requested handicapped license plates to cut down on the distance from her car to the supermarket, and she parked right near the door to her office, where she worked as a secretary for a consulting firm. She had given up teaching years ago.

Her children had noticed the change. On a shopping trip in the early evening, she'd often quit halfway through. It had reached a point where she no longer said she was tired. The kids would look at her, hold her arm, and say, "Time to go home."

Carolyn often fell asleep on the living room sofa early in the evening. And many nights she had woken up screaming in pain from leg cramps, caused by electrolyte imbalances. Through it all she remained dependent on the machine, tethered to it fifteen hours a week. She'd begun home dialysis two years before. That added flexibility, but it wore down Tom, who monitored the machine when she dialyzed herself late at night. Their lives had to be planned around the machine. For a significant number of people on dialysis, the restrictions, including those of food and liquid intake, become so overwhelming that they take their own lives. This was unthinkable to Carolyn. She pulled her own weight as a wife and mother, worked at her secretarial job, busied herself with knitting and needlepoint, and was an accomplished cook and gardener. But she realized that despite the extraordinary technology of hemodialysis, it did not function nearly as well as natural kidneys. On the day just before dialysis, the waste products in her bloodstream would build up to a high level, causing fatigue that was common to all dialysis patients. Now, that fatigue was dominating her life; she knew she was fading. She also knew that after years of waiting, her children were now more able to take care of themselves if she should not survive a transplant operation. The scales had finally tipped in favor of the transplant.

Carolyn's hospital room on the fourth floor of Walter Reed

was modern and efficient. She unpacked her small suitcase and put her belongings into the small vanity next to her bed and changed into her nightgown in the bathroom. She studied her face in the bathroom mirror, as if looking at the old version for the last time. Her skin had a dusty hue and her normally sharp features had softened, especially around her eyes, where the fluid retention showed most. She felt the omens were good for the transplant. She'd been dialyzed the night before and felt strong. She'd also had a blood transfusion two weeks earlier. She knew from Dr. Light that studies had shown that transplant patients who receive blood transfusions shortly before the transplant operation do better than those who do not. The reasons for this remain unclear. One theory is that the transfusion, and the transplant, both serve to overwhelm, and perhaps confuse, the immune system so that it is less likely to try to reject the implanted organ.

Carolyn stepped out of the bathroom as Tom was snapping her suitcase shut. He slid it into the closet and she slipped under the covers. An army major, Tom was an uncomplaining man with direct eyes and a strong build. They'd met as freshmen at the University of California. An Ohio native, he then transferred to West Point and they corresponded, met every summer, and were married on his graduation day. Although he made the military his career, he was in no way a rigid man. He spoke softly and laughed easily, and in many ways he was less strict with their children than Carolyn.

He reached over and held Carolyn's hand. "How are you doing?" he asked.

"Pretty good," she said.

"Anxious?" he asked.

"A little bit," she confessed.

She studied his face in the soft light of the room. She'd always loved his face. It was broad and open, with no trace of coyness; a masculine face, she thought. She was distressed that he seemed

59

to have aged ten years in the past two. Tom kept a lot inside himself, but Carolyn knew how hard her illness had been on him. He watched her on dialysis until one in the morning, and then got up at 5:30 A.M. for his job at the Pentagon. She also knew how deeply he'd been hurt recently when he learned he'd been "passed over," a military euphemism for being forced out of the service. Although the military didn't acknowledge it, ill dependents were sometimes a factor in these career decisions. He would officially leave the service in June, his twenty-year career at an end.

"I don't want you to come to the hospital every day. The kids need you a lot more than I do right now."

Tom understood. They'd talk on the telephone.

"I'm worried about Greg. He takes my illness so hard."

"I'll keep a close eye on him," Tom assured her.

"His grades slip and he gets so down. Linda can take care of herself, but Greg . . ."

"He'll do fine," Tom said. "We'll do things together and I'll try to keep his mind off it. And don't you keep worrying about us. You've got enough to handle right here."

A nurse came into the room and drew blood from Carolyn.

"Any idea when I'll be going to surgery?"

"Probably in a couple of hours," the nurse answered. "Have you talked to Dr. Light yet?"

"Just on the phone at home. He hasn't seen me here yet."

The nurse left. It was nearly 1 A.M.

Carolyn turned and looked directly at Tom. "I want you to know that no matter what happens, I'll never put you through home dialysis again. It was too much for all of us." She knew just how much he hated the machine, although he'd never complained about it.

"It was something we had to do," he said. "We got through it all right, even the electrical blackout."

60

In the more than twenty years of their marriage, they'd dealt with catastrophe and remained accepting people. Tom had married Carolyn knowing of her kidney problems.

Tom thought he should return home. Both of them sensed they were embarking on a new chapter in their lives. He leaned over and kissed Carolyn and squeezed her hand. "We're going to get through this," he said.

"I know we will," she answered.

"Take care," he said.

"You too."

Carolyn was alone. As positive as she tried to feel, she couldn't stop worrying about her children. Fears drifted in and out of her mind and she tried to turn them around. Think how overjoyed they would all be if this transplant succeeded and they could live a normal family life!

In the silence, she thought of the donor and her family. She understood the pain for which there is no solace. She tried to read a book, but couldn't concentrate. There were interruptions as doctors and nurses came by her room to talk with her. But mostly she dwelled in her own thoughts and waited, worried, and hoped.

It was late Sunday night and Kenneth Walsh heard the door to his room open. A voice spoke that was cheerful and female.

"Mr. Walsh?" the nurse asked.

He looked in the direction of her voice and saw only her indistinct outline against the light. "That's me," he said.

"Did one of the residents come by for your history earlier?"

"Yeah, young fellow was in tonight. I told him he didn't need to ask me anything. You must have a file a foot thick on me here."

"Come on now, it can't be all that bad."

" 'Fraid so. I'm a habitual offender."

61

Kenneth spoke like the true Bostonian he was. When he said "car" it came out "caaa," and "park" sounded like "pack." At sixty-eight his voice was gravelly, but still strong enough to shout for the Red Sox.

"Are you feeling all right?"

"Not bad for an old veteran of this place."

"Can I get you anything?"

"How about a shot of good whiskey?"

"That one's against the rules," she said.

"Figured you'd say that. Guess I'll stick to cigarettes. I'm entitled to one vice."

"One per customer," she said. "If you want a sleeping pill, call us."

"Will do," he said, "but I don't think I'll need one."

He stood up and walked around. He'd been in his room at the Massachusetts Eye and Ear Infirmary since 8 P.M., soon after he'd gotten a call that interrupted his work with his prized stamp collection. Despite his very poor sight, he was able to see his stamps with a high-powered magnifying glass, but he couldn't read. He'd always loved Ian Fleming and Helen MacInnes novels.

He turned on his radio and climbed back in bed to sleep and wait. He'd grown accustomed to waiting, and to disappointments. But he still was hopeful that this latest cornea could bring him sight. He'd asked about his donor when he first came in. It was a seventeen-year-old girl, they said, killed in a car accident. He shook his head. What a shame, he'd thought, someone that young.

Twenty-six years earlier, Kenneth was working as a draftsman. He'd drawn two long, parallel lines on his design sheet. When he stood back to look at them they appeared perfect. When he drew closer they converged into one, like railroad tracks coming together in the distance. He checked and rechecked; each time his eyes told him the lines came together as one. The cause of his vision distortion was juvenile cataracts, and that set off a series of events — including surgery that caused eye injury — that twelve years later led to glaucoma and finally to irreversible cornea damage.

His vision deteriorated to where he couldn't read newsprint. His distance vision was no better, and he had to quit driving and his work as a draftsman. In 1968 he received his first cornea transplant, but three months later it was rejected.

In 1970 his wife of more than twenty years died, leaving him on his own. This was followed by yet another eye problem, a detached retina in his right eye. The detachment was repaired and his vision improved, and because his need was so great, he continued to get transplants over the years. They were often rejected, but one worked so well for two years he could drive again, until it too was rejected.

Through it all he kept his spirits up and avoided dwelling on what life had dealt him. He had no children, but a number of relatives in the New England area remained close.

He wanted to work and at one time was a dishwasher at the Eye and Ear Infirmary. In recent years, as his sight worsened, he'd become less active. He lived in a pleasant rooming house, supported by his savings and social security.

Because he'd rejected ten corneas, he was an obvious candidate for the cornea-tissue-matching study. The previous fall he'd gone to Eye and Ear, just a few minutes from his Arlington home, where his blood was drawn and sent to Baltimore. Not surprisingly, he had an abundance of antibodies. That meant he was likely to reject tissue from other people. His name was added to the list in Dr. Stark's Johns Hopkins office to await the best-matched donor they could find, to try one more time to get sight for his right eye. It hadn't been good in ten years, since the retinal detachment.

Tomorrow would bring him one more chance.

～

It was 2 A.M. Monday in Cincinnati when the telephone rang in Jim and Betty Landis's home. Neither was asleep. It was Children's Hospital calling. The cross-match between Matthew and his donor kidney was completed, and it was a good one. The kidney had also arrived in excellent condition.

"When do you want me to bring Matthew in?" he asked.

"Can you be here by seven in the morning?"

"We'll be there," he said.

He hung up and turned to Betty. "It's go." Over the past few weeks they'd spent hours discussing this third transplant. They wondered at times whether they should put Matthew through the ordeal again if a kidney became available. Wouldn't it be more humane to accept what life dealt him and keep him the way he was for as long as they could? They remembered times when Matthew was so ill and so weakened by his transplant ordeals that they questioned their own motives for wanting him to live. They'd even thought he might be better off if he were taken from them. But their overriding impulse was to fight for life, and Matthew's survival so far proved he was a fighter too.

Betty walked to Matthew's bedroom. He was curled on his side, tucked under the covers, and deeply asleep. He clasped Curious George closely to his chest. Betty hadn't told him he might go back to the hospital, and he hadn't asked, but she and Jim knew he probably sensed he would. He drew long, deep breaths and Betty reached down and pulled his Superman comforter under his chin. She leaned over and kissed him, patted his head, and left the bedroom.

Back in her own bedroom, she and Jim slipped under the covers and Jim flicked off the light.

"I'll take him in tomorrow," Jim said.

"Are you scared?" she asked.

"Yeah."

"Me too."

"We'd be crazy not to be."

64

He put his arms around Betty and hugged her tightly to him. The pulls of the past three years caused them at times to almost become emotional strangers to one another, so much of them had gone into Matthew. Betty put her hand on Jim's hand and both lay quietly. They tried to sleep. Both knew it would be some time before they would be able to sleep easily again.

~~~~~~~~~~~~~~~~~~~~~~ FOUR

In January 1945, a young Boston woman was taken to Peter Bent Brigham Hospital suffering from an infection that within a short time caused her kidneys to shut down. Toxins built up in her blood over several days, and she lapsed into a coma. There was no kidney dialysis available, so her doctors watched helplessly as she slipped toward death.

Dr. Charles Hufnagel, a twenty-eight-year-old fellow who had performed animal organ transplants in Harvard University's surgical laboratories, heard about her case and was intrigued by it. He wondered if he could graft a donor kidney to this young woman that would last long enough for her kidneys to recover. He won the permission of the chief of medicine, largely because there was little risk since the woman was dying anyway. Hufnagel enlisted Dr. David Hume, a surgical resident, and within a short time they'd located a woman patient whose blood type matched the young woman's. Her family gave permission to remove her kidneys upon her death, which was imminent.

Because of the transplant's experimental nature, the hospital administration would not permit it to take place in the operating room, so Hufnagel and Hume made their own arrangements. Late that night, the donor died. One of her kidneys was removed immediately in the operating room, put in ice water, and rushed up to the dying woman's room on the hospital's second floor. There, under the light of two gooseneck lamps, Hufnagel attached the donor kidney to the dying woman's arm vessels. He draped a sterile dressing over the exposed kidney and kept it warm with the heat of the lamp. He rested the ureter on a towel, and within a few minutes urine began to be excreted as the kidney cleansed the blood that flowed through it. It kept working, and within two days the woman regained consciousness. Then her own kidneys began to function. At this time, Hufnagel removed the donor kidney, which had just begun to falter.

Although Hufnagel and Hume, both of whom enjoyed successful careers in organ transplantation over the next three decades, were jubilant over performing the first recorded human kidney transplant in history, news of it did not spread. The hospital feared criticism because of the highly unorthodox way the procedure was performed, and because there was no solid scientific basis for it at the time. So they kept it quiet and shared their milestone in silence.

Two weeks after their experiment, the young woman walked out of the hospital, and the first seed of human organ transplantation had been planted.

The transplantation of human organs blends both surgery and immunology: the first to implant the donor organ into the recipient's body, the second to modify and manipulate the body's attempts to reject it. Although great strides have been made since the quiet experiment at Peter Bent Brigham Hospital, organ transplantation still makes enormous demands on both the art and science of medicine. There often are no hard rules, tests, or pieces of elegant technology to tell a physician what to do in this very complicated field. Rather, it is where intuition, experience, and judgment blend with science.

At a little past 3:30 A.M. Monday, about three hours after Carolyn Blanchard had arrived at Walter Reed Army Medical Center, two orderlies came by to wheel her into surgery.

The kidney perfusion machine outside the fourth-floor operating room sent out a steady, rhythmic beep, like crickets on a summer night. Attached to the machine's tubing network was Lisa Kelly's left kidney. Fluid pumped through it to cool and nourish it.

At the scrub sink a few feet away, his hands and forearms covered with the foam of antibacterial soap, was Dr. Jimmy Light. In his early forties, tall, trim, and blond, he pressed the floor button and water ran up his arms, pushing any lingering bacteria away from his hands.

Carolyn lay on the operating table. Light's surgical team, accustomed to the odd hours of transplant surgery, was assembled and ready. Carolyn was draped and deeply anesthesized. Her eyes were taped shut to keep them moist and prevent abrasions to her corneas. The sound of her breathing was amplified by the passage of air and anesthetic gases through the tubes that led to her lungs. It echoed off the white ceramic tile covering the OR walls. Her abdomen was swabbed yellow with the antiseptic Betadine. Her heartbeat, blood pressure, and heart rate were displayed on digital monitors around the operating table. All were stable. Intravenous lines were already attached, pushing in immune-suppression drugs to ward off the rejection that would inevitably come.

Gowned and gloved, Light looked toward the anesthesiologist behind the drape that blocked his view of Carolyn's face.

"All set?" Light asked.

"Everything's ready," he answered.

The operating room was bright and warm, the smell of antiseptic strong. At 5:20 A.M. — thirty-three hours after Lisa Kelly's accident — Light made an opening incision along the lower right side of Carolyn's abdomen. The first transplant of Lisa Kelly's organs had begun.

Kenneth Walsh sat quietly in the wheelchair as it moved down the corridor toward his room. It was now Monday noon, and he'd spent three hours being examined. The retina and cornea specialists looked into his right eye with every instrument they had, but they couldn't agree on the cause of his poor sight. The retina specialists suspected the cornea, the cornea specialists the retina.

"There is no way to be certain," one of the doctors told him, "until we operate."

At a little after 2 P.M., a nurse came to Kenneth's room.

"We're going to take you to the OR in a few minutes."

"Guess I got everybody confused here. Maybe I'll make one of the medical journals."

The nurse handed him a pill and a glass of water.

"What is this going to do for me?" he asked.

"Just relax you."

Kenneth put the tranquilizer in his mouth and gulped it down with water.

"No reason to get all excited. Everything's out of my control now, anyway," he said.

"I'm sure everything's going to be fine."

"I hope so. When you've been around the track with this as many times as I have, about all you can do is hope."

A few minutes later, orderlies came to Kenneth's room, helped him onto the gurney, and wheeled him into the operating suite. In another operating room two doors away, Derrick Jackson lay deeply anesthetized, ready to receive Lisa Kelly's other cornea.

Dr. Kenneth Kenyon, head of the cornea service at the Eye and Ear Infirmary, sat just beyond Derrick's head, which rested firmly on a foam rubber pocket at the end of the operating table. He peered intently into the operating microscope that enlarged his field of vision fifteen-fold. Kenyon had taken a special interest in Derrick's case. As a Harvard medical student fifteen years earlier, he'd made a special study of the eye disease that had destroyed Derrick's corneas.

Because he could not see into Derrick's eye for the same reason Derrick could not see out of it, Kenyon had already performed ultrasound imaging to study the eye's inner structure. The image that was created on the oscilloscope showed that Derrick's inner eye was intact and healthy.

Clamps held Derrick's eye open, and Kenyon had carefully sutured the eye muscle to prevent the eye from moving. He lined up a small, circular instrument called a trephine over the center of Derrick's cornea. The trephine's sharp edge cut a ridge in the center of the cornea, much the way a cookie cutter does with dough. The cut was a precise circle, eight millimeters in diameter, in the only part of the cornea through which we see. With scissors, he cut the cornea section free and lifted it out with small forceps. A cornea is only a half to three-quarters of a millimeter thick, so Kenyon's margin for error was infinitesimally small.

The cornea transplant was not a new concept. The first recorded speculation about it was in 1789. The first animal experiment occurred in 1837 in Europe, when a surgeon successfully put the cornea of a dying gazelle into the blind eye of another gazelle. History does not record how successful that first transplant was. In 1846, general anesthesia was introduced, and human cornea transplants became possible. In 1872, the first animal-to-man experiment was attempted when a rabbit cornea was transplanted into a human, apparently with some temporary success. A number of similar experiments followed, but the corneas usually grew cloudy in a matter of weeks. The cause was probably infection, of which little was known during the nineteenth century.

In 1906, the first human cornea transplant using human donor tissue was reported in Austria. The recipient had suffered lye burns, and the graft came from the eye of a young boy who had lost it in an accident. That cornea graft apparently remained clear for a number of years, giving great hope for the procedure.

70

However, it wasn't until the 1950s that cornea transplantation came into wide use. A big reason was the establishment of eye banks that could supply corneas. Then in the 1960s and '70s, this operation made major strides when the operating microscope was developed. This permitted surgeons to have a much better view of the operating field. Also during this period, new, finer suture material came into use, along with other instrument advances, greatly increasing the success of cornea transplants.

Kenyon examined Lisa Kelly's clear, round cornea, which lay on a sterile block. He pressed the trephine against it and punched out a section called a corneal "button." It was identical in size to the one he'd just removed from Derrick's eye. It was washed with an antibiotic.

Although both of Derrick's corneas were damaged, Kenyon would only replace one. One reason was because of the shortage of corneas. Giving two people sight in one eye was preferable to giving one sight in both. But there was another reason. Because infection is a risk for cornea transplants, it was feared that if two cornea transplants were put in, and one became infected, the infection could spread to the other and both would be lost. Putting in only one reduced the chances for infection.

With forceps, Kenyon placed the cornea button from Lisa into the opening he'd made in Derrick's cornea and sewed it in place with sutures so fine they could not be seen by the naked eye, nor would they be felt by Derrick when he recovered. If the cornea can be compared to a watch crystal, then these neatly arranged sutures, when seen under a microscope, look like the watch's hour markers.

Kenyon then wove a final, uninterrupted suture around the cornea graft, cinched it up so it fit snugly, and took a final look through the microscope. The fit was perfect. He could now see the brown of Derrick's iris. It had taken Kenyon little more than an hour.

Waiting, always waiting, Jim thought as he and Betty sat on a sofa, as they had much of this Monday, in the first floor waiting room of Cincinnati's Children's Hospital. The room was spacious and well lighted, and the chapel adjoined it. Matthew had no infections, so the kidney transplant was still on.

Betty studied the face of Dr. John Noseworthy, the big bear of a man who sat across from her. Who'd ever think those huge hands could operate with such delicacy and precision inside little bodies? Noseworthy, who had only the faintest twang of his native Maine, spoke to them. It had become clear, he said, that Matthew's natural kidney was a continuing source of infection. It had caused the urinary tract infection that had canceled his transplant a month ago. With the immune-suppression drugs he'd be on for this transplant, even a mild infection could pose a grave risk.

Noseworthy then came to the point, which he knew would alarm Jim and Betty. "We want to take his kidney out when we do the transplant. I know it sounds sudden, but we've given it a lot of thought."

Noseworthy saw the surprise on Jim and Betty's faces. He couldn't offer statistical support, he said, it was a judgment call. It was also a potential trap. To increase Matthew's chances for a successful transplant meant they had to decrease his chances for survival if the transplant failed.

"What are the surgical risks?" Jim asked.

"There are some," Noseworthy said, "but the removal of his natural kidney shouldn't pose a much greater risk than the transplant operation itself."

Betty and Jim shifted uneasily on the sofa. Noseworthy realized they understood the implications of what he'd said very well. "This is a big decision," he said. "Why don't you talk it over and let me know."

They thanked him for talking with them and he left. Jim and

Betty were frightened at the thought of removing Matthew's kidney. As damaged as it was, it had kept him alive for three and a half years. His two previous kidney transplants had failed of hyperacute rejection within days of the surgery. If this one failed, Matthew had no safety net, and they weren't prepared for that.

They paced around the waiting room. "We've had some hard decisions to make," Jim said, "but this one beats them all."

He glanced over at Betty and read the worry and shock in her face; he knew his face showed the same thing. They prayed in the chapel, then came back to the waiting room. How can you make a decision like this for your child? Jim asked himself.

Betty cried softly. "I feel like picking him up and taking him home. Then at least we'd have him for a few months," she said.

They had nothing to go on but instinct, and Jim considered his own. "If it were me, I'd want the best chance I had at keeping the transplant. It's the only thing that'll give him a real chance at life."

Betty knew Jim was right; it was the only course that made sense.

Jim spoke again. "Matthew's got so much fight in him I think that's what he'd decide too. I think he'd want the whole thing or nothing at all."

"I know," Betty said, "I know."

Noseworthy came back to the waiting room for their answer. Matthew was due in the operating room soon.

Jim looked directly at Noseworthy. "Go ahead and take out his kidney. You have our permission."

Noseworthy told them he realized it was a hard decision to make, but it was the right one. "I'll do the best I can," he said. Jim and Betty walked to Matthew's room. There were only a few minutes left.

Matthew's toys were on the table by his bedside, and Curious George, propped up on the bed, was right next to him. They tried to hide their fears from Matthew. He'd grown silent and studied them as they explained what was going to happen.

"You're going to get a new kidney, Matthew," Betty said.

"I know," Matthew answered. His voice was soft, hardly audible.

"Mommy and Daddy are going to stay right here. We're not going to leave," Betty assured him.

Matthew understood, but still said nothing. At a little after 3 P.M., orderlies lifted him onto a stretcher and rolled him toward OR Three. Jim and Betty walked with him, holding his hands.

Betty spoke to him as she walked alongside. "We love you, honey. We'll be right here."

Matthew said nothing. He showed no fear, offered no complaints; only his eyes said he was scared. As his stretcher went through the swinging doors of the OR suite, Betty's and Jim's eyes filled, and they walked slowly back to the waiting room.

At a little after 4 P.M., with Matthew fully prepared for surgery, Noseworthy made the first incision into the lower right side of Matthew's abdomen. A transplanted kidney is not put toward the back, like a normal kidney. Rather, it is placed in the frontal abdominal area, where access to blood vessels and speed of surgery are greatly improved. Matthew's previous donor kidneys had been attached to his aorta and vena cava, the body's major blood vessels, because he'd been so small they were the only ones large enough to supply the kidneys with enough blood. Noseworthy didn't want to use these big vessels again. Now that Matthew was bigger, he wanted to attach Lisa's kidney to Matthew's right iliac artery and vein. After more than an hour's surgery through tissue made tough and fibrous by previous surgery, Noseworthy was astonished to find Matthew had no right iliac artery. His leg was supplied with blood from collateral vessels to compensate for his abnormality. Noseworthy quickly shifted to Matthew's left side.

Outside Jim and Betty tried small talk but soon gave up. How could they talk or think about anything else? They again went to the chapel and prayed, then came back to the waiting room. Hours had passed. At about 6 P.M., the waiting room door opened and they spun to look; it was a circulating nurse dressed in surgical greens. She smiled and spoke. "Dr. Noseworthy said to tell you things are going a little slowly, but everything is fine. Matthew is doing very well."

"That's good news," Jim said. "Thanks for taking the time to tell us."

"I'll give you another update later," she said.

It was difficult for Noseworthy to get his anatomical bearings at times because Matthew had so much fibrous tissue. Finally, he delicately exposed Matthew's left iliac vein and artery.

"Hemostat," he commanded.

A nurse slapped the special blood vessel clamp into his hand.

The vein was soft and pliable, and Noseworthy squeezed the hemostat to shut off its blood supply. The artery was tougher; it had the texture and strength of frozen clothesline rope. He squeezed another hemostat and closed off its blood flow.

"I'm ready for the kidney," Noseworthy announced.

The circulating nurse detached Lisa's kidney from the tubing of the perfusion machine, wrapped it in a sterile towel, and carried it across the OR to Noseworthy.

He took it in his hand, flushed it with saline solution, and gently placed it in the small pocket he'd fashioned in Matthew's abdomen. The kidney was the size of a small fist, and it was purplish blue in color. Then Noseworthy made precisely angled cuts in Matthew's iliac artery and vein so he could attach them to the renal vessels from Lisa's kidney. This attachment of one blood vessel to another is called anastomosis, and until the turn of the century it was considered an impossible surgical feat. The

French surgeon who first accomplished it was awarded the Nobel Prize in Medicine.

As Noseworthy began sewing the vessels together — the most important part of the surgery — he glanced at the clock. He wanted to finish within thirty minutes to lessen any risk of harm to the kidney. He meticulously wove stitch after stitch, each a millimeter from the one before it. There was no tolerance for error. If the anastomosis was flawed, and that flaw went undetected, the kidney could be lost.

His huge hands worked quickly and precisely. Demands for instruments grew sharper; concentration became absolute.

"How much time?" he asked without looking up.

"Eleven minutes," a nurse answered.

He kept weaving the curved suturing needle. It looked like a tiny, barbless fishhook. He slid it into Lisa's vein, then looped it into Matthew's, then pulled it out with small forceps, then repeated it. Each stitch strengthened the bond between Lisa's kidney and Matthew.

"How much time?"

"Fourteen minutes," the nurse answered.

The artery, about the size and shape of a pencil, was tougher. He pushed the needle harder, stitch after stitch.

"How much time?"

"Twenty-three minutes," the nurse answered.

Noseworthy's neck and shoulders were tight from the tension. Now, with the final stitch, the vessels were tied to one another as tightly as a weld. Noseworthy looked up at the clock. It had taken exactly thirty minutes.

Now came the test of his work, and the test of the kidney. First Noseworthy released the clamp on the vein. The blood, under much less pressure here than in the artery, flowed from Matthew into Lisa's kidney. Noseworthy examined the anastomosis for leaks.

76

"Looks good," he said.

Now the harder test. He released the clamp from Matthew's iliac artery. Like a bursting dam, Matthew's blood rushed into Lisa's kidney. Nothing came closer to the creation of life itself than seeing that shrunken, discolored donor kidney swell and throb as life-giving blood poured into it. The kidney turned pink and healthy. Then small drops of urine trickled out of the ureter and onto a sterile towel.

"It's making urine!" a nurse yelled. Muffled cheers were heard under the surgical masks around the operating table. The kidney worked.

It had been almost forty-eight hours to the minute since Lisa Kelly's accident.

Noseworthy now attached the ureter from Lisa's kidney to Matthew's bladder, and then moved toward the back to get out his natural kidney. Once Noseworthy saw it he understood why it had caused Matthew so much trouble. It was mottled and shrunken, and on it were patches of gray scarring, all signs of chronic infection. It was a wonder it had worked at all.

The total time in the OR had been eight and a half hours. Noseworthy could feel the fatigue in his legs and back, but he was exhilarated that the entire operation had gone so well. Matthew was resilient, his vital signs had remained strong and stable.

It was just after 11 P.M. when Matthew was wheeled from the OR to the isolation section of the intensive care unit on the fourth floor. He was immune-suppressed from the intravenous drugs given him during surgery. Noseworthy, still in his scrub suit, met Jim and Betty.

"It looks very good," he said. "The kidney pinked up beautifully."

Relief enveloped Jim and Betty. Noseworthy explained the problem with the iliac artery and told them the natural kidney was in bad condition and it was wise to remove it. They were gratified. Noseworthy, his face a picture of exhaustion, moved to leave.

Jim called to him and reached out his hand. "Thank you, doctor."

Noseworthy smiled, shook his head approvingly, and headed for the surgeon's locker room.

Jim and Betty took an elevator to the intensive care unit. They put on sterile masks and gowns. Once Betty spotted Matthew's bed she moved immediately toward him. He was still groggy from anesthesia. She had seen him like this many times in his young life, and every time it broke her heart.

They stood over his bed, and Betty reached down and took his tiny hand in hers. She squeezed it gently and kneeled next to him. "We're here, Matthew, Mommy and Daddy are here," she whispered over and over. Matthew stirred slightly, but could not say anything.

They stayed for several minutes, until one of the nurses said it would be better if they left for now. Betty let go of Matthew's hand, and they returned to the waiting room, where they took turns sleeping and visiting Matthew throughout the night.

PART II

THE NEXT TWENTY-FOUR MONTHS

≈≈≈≈≈≈≈≈≈≈≈≈ F I V E

The line of young people extended beyond the long canopy outside the funeral home. The boys, dressed in suits and sport coats, tugged uncomfortably at their ties and tight collars. The girls wore dresses and long coats. They spoke in whispers to one another as the line shifted forward slowly on this sunny Tuesday afternoon.

The Kelly family was inside, in a room that was dark and heavy, the sounds absorbed by the thick carpeting and drapes. Maureen stood next to her mother, touching her shoulder at times, while keeping her eye on her father. They all felt numb, as if everything that was happening wasn't quite real.

Maureen watched as Joanne, the young girl with Lisa the night of the accident, walked hesitantly through the front door. The sight of her startled Maureen. It was as if her presence was a sharp reminder of Lisa's death. Joanne moved toward the Kellys, but couldn't bring herself to walk up and talk to them. Instead, her mother did.

"I'm so sorry," she said to Louise. "Joanne is so distraught she can't even talk."

Louise said she understood and thanked Joanne's mother for coming.

A young boy, tall and dark-haired, lingered near the Kellys. His name was Raymond and Louise recognized him. He had taken Lisa out a few times, and although they hadn't had a romance, they had become close friends. He was a very good young artist.

He approached Louise uneasily and spoke. "I used to give Lisa some of my pictures."

"Yes, she told us, Raymond," Louise said. "They were beautiful pictures, and she treasured them."

Raymond nodded and walked off. As Maureen watched Lisa's classmates, she thought of the times she and Lisa had talked of the future. Lisa had said she might like to work with children, perhaps as a teacher. Maureen felt an ache thinking about it now.

Maureen watched Ellen standing off to the side talking quietly with a small group of young people. Even when she and Lisa had fought, more often than not their fights had dissolved into laughter. And when they were younger, Lisa had often ended them by putting her arms around Ellen and embracing her. Ellen had spent most of the time since Lisa's death in her room, alone. She still had not talked of Lisa's death, and her expression was almost empty of emotion, except for her eyes. They had the look of a wounded animal, hurt and afraid. Everything else seemed locked up inside her, and that worried Maureen and her mother.

These thoughts were jarred when a poorly dressed man moved through the line of students and announced, "I'm her real daddy." The Kellys recognized him as Lisa's real father, although they hadn't seen him in years.

He first approached Eugene Kelly, who regarded him as a man with minimal opportunities in life. Eugene spoke pleasantly to him, and the man then approached Maureen, who was cordial as well. He smiled awkwardly and approached Ellen, but she shrank away from him. He stayed for a few more minutes, but spoke to no one else. Then he walked out.

He'd learned of Lisa's death from a priest the Kellys knew,

the same one who had visited Lisa and Ellen's mother at the mental hospital to break the news.

"What did she say when you told her, Father?" Louise had asked.

"She didn't show any emotion," the priest had answered, "and she didn't say a word about Lisa. She acted as if she didn't understand a word I said."

Louise almost envied her.

That evening, after the wake, they all had supper at Louise's house. Maureen was worried that cooking for everyone might be too much for her mother.

"I'd like to. It'll keep me busy," Louise told her.

After dinner, they all returned to the funeral home as another group of mourners came by to pay their respects. No one in the Kelly family had slept much since Saturday night, but they didn't feel tired as they stood once again in the small receiving line.

Maureen realized Lisa's death, and the sudden visit of the father she hadn't seen in years, stirred many painful emotions in Ellen. She'd grown even more withdrawn in the past few hours. They had assured her that Lisa's death would not change their adoption plans. Ellen said she realized that; no reassurance was necessary.

By 9 P.M., all the funeral-home visitors had left. Maureen watched as Ellen moved slowly toward Lisa's closed casket. She reached out to touch it, as if making a final contact with her sister. Maureen walked slowly over to her.

"I know how badly you hurt, I'm hurting too," Maureen whispered.

Ellen nodded, but said nothing. Maureen put her arm around Ellen and held her tightly, and Ellen put her arm around Maureen. Both stood silently for several moments, looking at Lisa's casket.

It was late in the afternoon and the sky outside was dark gray. Jo Leslie reached behind the bottles of perfusion fluid and took a diet cola from the refrigerator located in the small laboratory adjacent to her office. She flipped open the top and walked back to her desk. She was alone in the office. It felt stuffy and over-heated, so she wedged open a window and took a deep breath of cold air. She looked over the pile of papers on her desk. She discarded some, filed others, and put a couple in the middle of her desk to remind herself to look them over more carefully tomorrow. Much time was absorbed in the paperwork of organ transplantation, forms, bills, letters. It never seemed to stop. The work was relentless.

She was physically tired from the long hours she'd put in over the last few days. She'd been authorized to hire a third pro-curement person for her office. She'd chosen a nurse named Fran Danella, who would start very soon. But for the past several weeks, she and Bob Grant had had to do most everything, and it was catching up with her. Sixty- and seventy-hour work weeks were routine, and she'd already accumulated a total of nearly two hundred hours of overtime since the beginning of the year.

The morning had been difficult in another way. A nurse had called her at 11 A.M. to alert her to a potential donor in Shock-trauma. Once there, Jo discovered it was a young man with a history of psychiatric problems. He'd suffered an irreversible brain injury from a fall, and it wasn't certain if it was accidental or self-inflicted.

Jo went to the small waiting room and met the family. They hardly acknowledged her when she introduced herself. A brother, dressed in jeans and dark jacket, showed no outward emotion, except anger. A sister sat on a small sofa, repeating, "Why did he do this to us?" The mother, a graying, gaunt woman in her late fifties, sat and stared blankly. Her face was a mask. Her minister was at her side.

84

Jo expressed her sorrow to them and brought up the idea of organ donation.

"I'd like you to consider it for yourselves," she said.

There were several moments of silence before the mother spoke. "He never wanted anyone to touch him," she said.

In all her dealings with families, Jo never tried to coerce them or press them with guilt by telling them she had someone waiting who desperately needed an organ. Her job wasn't to make life harder for the families. So she told the mother only that he would not feel any pain if she decided on donation, and gave them all the room they needed to make up their minds.

The mother told Jo she wanted to think it over. Jo left and walked to Neurotrauma to make certain that if the answer was yes, which she doubted, everything was in order to go ahead with the donation.

She thought how different this family was from the Kellys. The only emotions she'd felt from this one were anger and detachment; there was no sense of grief or sorrow for the victim, as was so clear with the Kellys.

A few minutes later, the minister found Jo. "The family wanted me to tell you that they decided against organ donation," he said.

"Could I speak to them?" Jo asked. "I just want to make them comfortable with that decision."

The minister led her back. Jo knelt at the mother's side. "Every family's decision is right for them, and you should not feel bad for turning me down," she said. She again said how sorry she was. The mother nodded, but said nothing, and Jo moved to leave.

It was now 6:30 P.M. Jo finished her soda and locked up the office, and twenty minutes later she was home. She showered, got into her nightgown, and read in bed for a while. Again she thought of the Kellys. Some families stayed with her, and she knew the Kellys would be one of them. She wondered how they were doing. Tomorrow she'd write them a letter to thank them for their generosity, and to tell them something of the four people they'd helped. She also wanted to tell them she'd taken Lisa's adrenal glands to Dr. Hugo Moser, an internationally recognized researcher at Johns Hopkins. Dr. Moser was using the adrenals for research into a disease called adreno-leuko-dystrophy. Jo hoped her letter would let the Kellys understand the scope of their gift, and help begin the long process of healing.

It was 8 A.M. and cold for mid-March as Paul McEnery aimed his battered Volkswagen bug, the one he called the "yellow Cadillac," into his accustomed parking place behind the brick and granite buildings of Cincinnati Children's Hospital. He grabbed his worn leather briefcase and headed toward the Research Foundation Building. He took long, loping strides across the parking lot. A native of Chicago, he was accustomed to cold winters.

His fourth-floor office was cluttered with boxes of bumper stickers, pledge cards, buttons, tee shirts, and other paraphernalia used to raise money for the Ronald McDonald house, a residential hotel for out-of-town parents of sick children. McEnery headed the local drive to build this facility.

He walked to the doctors' lounge, poured himself a cup of coffee, and stopped by the office of Monica Quinlan, the nephrology nurse and key assistant.

"How's everyone doing today?" he asked.

Monica, a bubbly woman in her twenties, handed him a clipboard holding the overnight patient status reports.

"How's Matthew?" McEnery asked.

"Looks like the beginning of some rejection," Monica answered.

McEnery took the status reports to his desk and sipped coffee as he studied them. A pediatrician who specialized in kidney disease, McEnery was keenly interested in Matthew's progress and remembered the hard disappointments he'd been through. McEnery also realized Matthew was not quitting in the face of his illness. He'd seen him fight back, even when they'd almost given up hope. Because Matthew's two earlier transplants had been rejected so quickly and violently, now only five days since his transplant the mildest sign of rejection was worrisome. Rejection was expected because every transplanted organ experiences some.

The first clear evidence of how serious an obstacle rejection was for human organ transplants had surfaced more than thirty years earlier, in 1950, when Ruth Tucker, a forty-nine-year-old Chicago housewife, underwent the first human kidney transplant in which a donor kidney was placed inside the body to permanently replace diseased kidneys. For decades, organ transplants had tantalized medical researchers, but the experience with Mrs. Tucker showed that what seemed simple in concept — replacing a damaged organ with a healthy one — was profoundly difficult in execution.

Dr. Richard Lawler, a Chicago surgeon, had suggested the transplant to Mrs. Tucker. She agreed because kidney dialysis was still highly experimental and there were no machines available to replace her failing kidneys. The surgery succeeded. It generated headlines throughout the country, and the patient did well for a number of months. Then her urine output declined markedly. Dr. Lawler re-operated to find the source of the problem and discovered to his surprise that the transplanted kidney was gone. After a careful search, he found a small, shrunken remnant of what once was the kidney. It had been virtually devoured by the immune system. Mrs. Tucker survived four more years on the remaining function in her other kidney, but died when that one failed.

McEnery believed Matthew's immune system, which saw the donor kidney as a foreign invader, was rejecting the kidney in the same way Ruth Tucker's immune system had, by attacking it with millions of antibodies carried to the kidney by the bloodstream. Over the years, many methods were tried to prevent this attack. Whole-body radiation suppressed the immune response and was given to a number of early transplant recipients. So were bone-marrow transfusions. Both methods helped lessen rejection, but they also exposed the patients to serious risks and often caused their immunity to completely vanish. This left them defenseless against illness. More refined techniques were needed, and in the late 1950s and early 1960s, special drugs were developed that blocked immune response. This did not solve the problem of rejection, but it gave the patients, and the donor organ, a better chance at survival.

McEnery slipped on his white lab coat and stopped to pick up Monica.

They took the elevator to the basement and proceeded through a long tunnel-like corridor that connected the research foundation to the main hospital. A collection of residents and nephrology fellows, along with McEnery and Monica, headed toward Two East, where Matthew was in his room, isolated from other patients.

McEnery was a low-key, plain-speaking man who was widely regarded as one of the country's outstanding pediatric kidney specialists. He was in his midforties and lived modestly in an old Cincinnati neighborhood with his wife and two young daughters. His older daughter had a kidney problem that worried him, and he was no stranger to disease himself. He'd been an insulin-dependent diabetic since his early college days.

For most of the young patients he cared for, kidney disease was a chronic problem. That meant he knew them for long periods of time, just as he'd known Matthew. He grew to care about many of them, as he'd grown to care deeply about Matthew. It sometimes made professional detachment difficult. Some physicians could not tolerate the emotional wear and tear of pediatric kidney disease. Despite the gratification of guiding young patients through medical crises and on to normal lives, they could not accept the losses and suffering of these young people. Many left the field. The losses hurt McEnery too, and he protected himself against them as best he could. He attended the weddings and graduations of his patients, but never the funerals.

Because Cincinnati Children's Hospital was in the forefront of pediatric kidney transplants, much of McEnery's time was spent with children during the difficult post-transplant period. The children came to Cincinnati from all over the Midwest. McEnery and his colleagues believed strongly in transplanting children with failed kidneys as early as possible. He'd helped compile evidence that successful kidney transplants before the age of six meant children could grow normally. The doctors at Children's also emphasized unrelated donors — instead of family donors — more than most other transplant centers. This diminished the chances of the transplant succeeding because tissue matching was not as good, but it improved the psychological risks. Some patients suffered guilt and depression when they rejected a family member's kidney, and some family donors became angry when the recipient lost the kidney.

Jim and Betty had never considered one of their daughters for kidney donorship because they did not want to burden them with psychological or physical risks, but they had offered themselves after Matthew's second rejection. By then he'd grown enough so he could accept an adult-sized kidney. But cross-matching tests by the lab showed Matthew would reject a kidney from either of them. His prior transplants and blood transfusions had apparently created antibodies that would attack tissue from his own parents. It was another in the long list of disappointments Jim and Betty had suffered.

McEnery's voice was cheerful as he entered Matthew's room. "Hello, Matthew. How you feeling today? Good, I hope."

Lying in bed with Curious George right next to him, Matthew

stared at McEnery with expressionless eyes. He often grew silent in the hospital, sometimes only speaking to Betty. He would not speak at all amid a large gathering.

Jim Landis stood next to the doctors. "I don't think you're going to get Matthew to say much this morning," Jim said.

"That's not unusual," McEnery said, smiling.

Matthew clutched at Curious George as McEnery leaned over and palpated his new kidney. He was happy to feel sharp, defined edges, a sign that the rejection hadn't softened it.

"Still feels very healthy," McEnery announced.

"That hurt you, Matthew?" Monica asked.

There was still no answer from Matthew.

Jim spoke. "He's felt a little pain, but he hasn't complained much."

"Well," McEnery said, "he's not much of a complainer anyway. Are you, Matthew?" Matthew just looked up at him.

On the status report McEnery held were the two, unmistakable signs of rejection. One was the rise in Matthew's serum creatinine leavel. Creatinine is a waste product of protein metabolism. If Matthew's kidney were perfectly healthy, his creatinine level would measure less than one, perhaps .4 or .5. But the reading was 1.4, too high.

The second number that concerned McEnery was BUN, blood urea nitrogen. The amount of this waste product in the blood was a measure of the kidney's ability to rid the body of wastes, one of its major functions. Matthew's BUN level was more than double normal. Matthew was taking two drugs that fought rejection in different ways. Imuran sought to disguise his donor kidney as a natural part of him, while Prednisone, a steroid, diminished the immune system's ability to attack. Both appeared to be falling short. It was a situation that demanded a strong, immediate response.

McEnery spoke to Jim. "I'm going to put him on Solu-Medrol." Jim knew that Solu-Medrol, an immune suppressant, was a very potent steroid that always had the potential for serious side effects.

There are three types of rejection: hyperacute, acute, and chronic. Matthew's was the acute type, which was the most treatable. His first two kidney transplants had suffered hyperacute rejections. These were so overwhelming that no drugs available to the doctors could stop them from destroying the kidneys. The other type of unstoppable rejection was chronic. This is a slow process that may take months to destroy the donor kidney, but which also cannot be stemmed by immune-suppression drugs.

McEnery was confident they'd caught this rejection episode early, but the treatment for it was always a tightrope. If too strong, Matthew would be wide open to infections. A simple cold, which a normal three-year-old could throw off in a few days, would be very risky. If the immune suppression was too weak, it invited the antibodies to destroy his kidney. Rejections could occur at any time, and just because one was turned back didn't mean another wasn't on the way. It was an often confusing battle that sometimes put the survival of the kidney and the survival of the patient in opposition. Judgment and experience on the part of the doctors were always critical.

McEnery was optimistic about Matthew. He hoped the third time might be the charm, even though there was only a 50-50 statistical chance Matthew would still have this kidney in a year's time. He knew if Matthew kept the kidney for a year, it would settle down, become a part of him. Then it could stay with him for a long time, even into early adulthood, perhaps for a full lifetime. No one could predict. Each day was another step closer to that year.

McEnery wrote his order into Matthew's chart and looked down at him and smiled. "I'll come by and see you a little later, okay, Matthew?"

Matthew still didn't speak.

They had to keep daily track of Matthew's kidney-function numbers, and that meant a blood sample every morning. Monica was the one person who could stick a needle into Matthew without causing tears. His eyes brightened whenever he saw her.

Now that the doctors had left, Monica approached. "Hi, Matthew. How are you doing?"

Matthew would speak now, but only through Curious George. "I ask George," he replied. Monica smiled and waited.

"George say he feel a little tired," Matthew said.

Monica couldn't help having favorites, and Matthew was hers.

"I have to take a little blood," she said. "Is that okay with George?"

Matthew turned to George. "George say he won't cry."

"George is very brave," Monica answered. She pretended to take blood from Curious George, and when she finished she put a Band-Aid on George's arm.

"There now, that should take care of George."

"George and me don't cry," he said.

Monica then carefully inserted the needle into Matthew's arm and drew enough blood to run the kidney-function tests.

"That didn't hurt too much, did it, Matthew?"

Matthew's eyes were still closed and his fists clenched. "No . . . not much," he said.

Monica patiently played out this game every time she took blood from Matthew. She had come to realize that Curious George was, in some way at least, Matthew's sick self. It was the part of him he knew was ill but wanted to keep separate from himself.

"Bye-bye," she said. "See you later."

"George say goodbye," Matthew called to her.

Jim remained in Matthew's hospital room after Monica left.

He asked Matthew if he wanted anything. Matthew shook his head no. Matthew wouldn't talk now.

Jim was tired, but not just from the vigils at the hospital these past few days. He'd gone beyond the point of exhaustion a long time ago. He'd set himself a goal three months earlier to finish four tasks: build shelves in his garage, build a jungle gym for the kids, fix the transmission on his sister's car, and repair his truck. Normally it would have taken a couple of weeks of spare time to do all four. All he'd done so far was build one half of the shelves. After he got off work every night he went to bed around 3 A.M., slept four or five hours, and rushed off to the hospital to be with Matthew during the morning and early afternoon. He did it every day.

Now he sat next to Matthew's bed, quietly watching him. Matthew often had bouts with high blood pressure, a common problem in victims of kidney disease, and Jim and Betty had found they often could lower it just by comforting him.

Matthew pressed his hands together and placed them under his face, which had grown moon-shaped from the steroid drugs. He lay on his side, sometimes sleeping, sometimes just staring with his big, brown eyes. Jim asked him if he wanted him to turn on the television set. Getting no response, he wondered what Matthew thought about in these deep silences.

After a nap, Matthew sat up in bed. "I want to paint now," he announced.

Jim fetched his poster paints, which were kept in an empty egg carton near his bedside. Matthew dipped the brushes into the brightest colors and splashed the colors on paper. Yellows blended with bright reds in large, formless patterns.

"Very good, Matthew, I like that," Jim said as Matthew painted.

Matthew had always been able to amuse himself for long periods of time, perhaps because of his nature, perhaps because he'd had to. He painted for nearly two hours, and Jim hung up his new creations in his room. It was nearly afternoon and Jim had to leave for work.

"Time for me to go, Matthew," Jim said. "Mommy will be here in a little while."

Matthew said nothing. He just kept watching Jim.

"Kiss goodbye?" Jim asked, leaning over.

He reached around and hugged his son and Matthew still didn't say a word. Then Matthew reached his small arm around Jim's back and hugged him and patted him, as if to say, It's okay, Dad, it's going to be okay.

Two days later the numbers told the good news: the rejection was beaten. Plans were made for Matthew to go home soon.

SIX

T he Lord came into my life when I was drinking and smoking and doing a lot of bad stuff . . . but all that's behind me now. I don't do that no more."

Each statement was quickly punctuated with a chorus of "Amen, brother," or "Praise the Lord," as Derrick, dressed in blue jeans and a plaid shirt, stood before the small congregation, giving his "testimony." He had been moved to speak, and now that he'd begun, inspiration seemed to take over. More and more he became caught up in his message and his usual reticence melted, replaced by a strong, emotional voice. He paced in front of the wooden cross as everyone watched.

"I had cornea transplants before . . . but the Lord wasn't in my life then. . . . I was in the world . . . and I lost the corneas . . . but that's changed now."

"Praise God," a man's voice cried out.

"One doctor even told me I didn't deserve another cornea because I never took care of the ones I had before. . . . That was true before the Lord came into my life . . . but not this time."

"Praise Jesus," a woman called out.

"I know the Lord gave me this cornea . . . this chance to see again. . . . I know you all prayed for me. . . . I don't know why He did it . . . I know it meant He had to take someone else's life. . . . I don't know His plan . . . but I know I want

95

to do His work. . . . Now that He has come into my life, I want to serve Him."

"Praise God . . . Praise God," several voices again shouted.

"Sometimes in my life I got real angry 'cause my eyes failed. But maybe if I'd had healthy eyes and gone into the world and made a lot of money, maybe I'd have never found the Lord and I still would be blind."

"Hallelujah!"

Derrick finished his testimony, bowed his head, and walked slowly back to his pew and sat down next to Shirley. The congregation then began to sing a hymn. It was a week to the day since Derrick's brother had come to this little church to find him. He had been discharged from the Massachusetts Eye and Ear Infirmary on Friday and Shirley had driven him home. He had felt compelled to tell his church members of the experience, how God made it possible.

When the service ended, fellow church members came up to Derrick and surrounded him, shook his hand, hugged him. They were young and old, black and white, all joined by their genuine feeling for Derrick and the "miracle" they'd witnessed. Slowly he pulled away from everyone and he and Shirley began to gather up her three children. They all walked to Shirley's car in the church parking lot and she drove Derrick home. Derrick had an appointment the next day at the Eye and Ear Infirmary. Shirley told him she'd pick him up at the bus station when he returned from Boston.

Late the next morning, Derrick sat alone in a small examining room of the Massachusetts Eye and Ear Infirmary, awaiting Dr. Kenyon. He had a noon appointment and he'd arrived a half hour early. On the wall near the door was an eye chart; to the back of the room was a slit lamp, used by ophthalmologists to see inside the eye. On the desk in front of him was his file. Without looking in it, Derrick knew there was a lot of negative information in there about his missed appointments and failure to comply with directions. Part of my old life, he thought to himself.

He heard the door swing open and looked up to see Dr. Kenyon's smiling face. Kenyon was in his early forties. He was upbeat and friendly, and had told Derrick at the outset that he would hold nothing in his past against him.

"How've you been feeling, Derrick?" he asked.

"Pretty good. No complaints," Derrick answered.

"Is that your Bible?" Kenyon asked.

"Yeah, I carry it everywhere."

"Never got past the pictures, myself," Kenyon kidded. Then he paused. "Are you actually reading already?"

"I've been reading for a few days now," Derrick answered.

Kenyon was incredulous. "Can I take a look at it?"

"See for yourself," Derrick said.

It was a large-print Bible, but Kenyon was surprised that Derrick could read anything this soon after the transplant.

"You're making remarkable progress," Kenyon told him.

Kenyon examined Derrick's eye. There was no sign of infection or rejection. Derrick assured him he'd faithfully put in his antibiotic eye drops.

"I expect the vision to clear more and more within the next several weeks," Kenyon said.

"I'm patient," Derrick told him.

Kenyon asked him to make an appointment to come back in a month, and left.

As Kenyon walked away, he thought to himself that he'd never seen a patient respond so quickly and so well to a cornea transplant.

Derrick's remarkable progress had much to do with Kenyon's skill, the excellent quality of Lisa Kelly's cornea, and Derrick's care of it. But probably there were other reasons. His prior transplants came before he found Shirley, and religion. Before, he'd been consumed with anger and disappointment. It's been shown in many studies that negative emotions appear to impair the immune system and the healing process, leaving us vulnerable to disease, and that positive emotions, such as happiness, laughter, and love, can aid our physical well-being.

Also, there is reasonable evidence that by believing you will get well — sometimes called "the placebo effect" — you can help healing. Sometimes this belief can overcome enormous medical obstacles.

Derrick now enjoyed the happiest time of his young life. He had found a woman who cared about him. He had found religion, and he believed in its power. Because of this, Derrick's own mind may have become his greatest healer.

When Kenyon had first removed the bandages from his eye the day after the transplant surgery, it was a transcendent moment for Derrick. Images were hazy, but heads had faces, doors and windows had sharply defined shapes. He lay there, hardly hearing the conversation, lost in his own joy. Now, as he walked up Charles Street toward the bus station, the miracle of sight came back to him in smaller ways. The faces that came toward him were grim and unsmiling, yet Derrick reveled in the uniqueness of each. He crossed the street unassisted, without the fear of the unseen.

The sight that stayed with him most was his first clear view of Shirley's face. He'd seen it the day she came to Boston to drive him home after the cornea transplant. He'd known her as a spiritual, caring person, but he hadn't realized she was pretty until his first glimpse of her as she walked into his room. Up to now, they'd shared a deepening friendship, but not a romance. Derrick had felt unappealing to women ever since a girl he'd liked in high school had told him she didn't want to go out with him. He asked her why, and she was brutally honest. "Your eyes," she said. "I just can't stand to look at them."

Shirley met him at the Springfield bus terminal, and they walked to her car and drove into the early rush-hour traffic. A few minutes later Shirley pulled up in front of Derrick's home, a second-floor walk-up in a working-class section of West Springfield.

"I guess you've probably noticed me staring at you lately," Derrick said.

"Oh, a little bit," Shirley answered. In fact, she'd noticed it a lot.

"Well, I've been doing it because you're so pretty."

Shirley laughed. "I was hoping it wasn't because you were so disappointed now that you could see what I looked like."

Derrick was embarrassed. "Oh, no, not at all. Just the opposite."

They both laughed from embarrassment. Then they leaned toward one another and embraced. Finally, Shirley eased away. "I've got to get home to the kids," she said. "Do you want to come over for dinner tomorrow night?"

"That sounds great," Derrick replied, and then he walked up to his apartment.

It was a late March morning and the sun glistened on the dampened street below Kenneth Walsh's rooming house. He heard the distant rush of cars and the voices of young children on their way to school. He parted the sheer white curtain and looked out. He saw the street — and the world — through a small hole. It was like peering through a knothole at a baseball game, he thought.

After all the debate among the doctors as to the causes of his right eye problem, the cornea transplant answered it. The more serious problem was an irreparable macula fold, caused by his earlier retinal detachment. The cornea transplant worked perfectly, but because of the macula fold, Walsh's sight would never get beyond looking through that knothole. He still felt the ache of his disappointment.

Dressed in gray slacks and a tan cardigan sweater, he walked to his kitchenette. He was running low on groceries. He put on some hot water for instant coffee. After he gulped that down, he moved downstairs and edged toward the door. He met Mrs. Cooper, his landlady, who was sweeping the steps. She was in her late fifties, a stocky, cheerful woman who had turned her old home into a boardinghouse after the death of her husband two years earlier.

"How you feeling today, Mr. Walsh?"

"Oh, not bad for an old-timer."

"Your eye doing better?"

"About the same. No big changes."

"It takes time," she said.

"Yes," he said, but he knew time would never improve the sight in his right eye. His doctors were certain of that, and so was he. He never showed his disappointment or uttered a word of self-pity, nor would he. With great effort, he could still work on his stamp collection. It just took a long time with the magnifying glass. He could also listen to the radio and feel the warmth of a sunny day.

"Be back in a little bit," he called to Mrs. Cooper. He extended his white cane, moved slowly down the steps, and walked along the sidewalk toward the grocery store.

Carolyn Blanchard stared at her hands. They had been deeply ridged, the skin wrinkled and yellow. They'd distressed her for years. They'd been the worn-out hands of an old woman. Now she held them out in front of her and turned them slowly in the soft light, as if she were examining a new manicure. She marveled at the change. The color was a healthy flesh tone, the wrinkles had disappeared.

She'd sensed another change — a deep, internal cleansing that seemed to purify her body. She'd spent the first few days in the hospital watching the bladder catheter carrying urine from her body and she'd told Tom, "I guess I'm one of the few people in the world who would get so much joy from watching that."

It was now late March, three weeks since her transplant. She'd been released from the hospital two weeks to the day after surgery, and had sailed through the postoperative period spectacularly. By the third day after surgery, she'd felt stronger than she'd felt in years. When Dr. Light came to see her a few days after he'd put in the kidney, she said, "I never believed I could feel this well again."

Now as Carolyn sat at her kitchen table, with Linda and Greg off at school and Tom at work, her feeling of well-being made the sun streaming through the window look brighter to her, and the early Washington spring more glorious than she'd ever remembered. The daffodils lining her backyard fence were in bloom; so were the forsythia bushes.

She poured herself a big glass of orange juice. Dr. Light had told her to drink plenty of fluids, a complete reversal of her time on dialysis when fluid intake was extremely limited. She gulped it down. A month earlier that would have been unthinkable, perhaps even fatal. With no kidneys, that much potassium could have caused electrical disturbances in her heart.

She walked to her bathroom and stepped on the scale. She had lost eighteen pounds, most of it from fluid. Her new kidney was far more efficient at removing fluid from her body than the dialysis machine. She could see she appeared more rested. She'd even noticed changes in Tom. On the drive home from Walter Reed, he'd confessed to her just how much he hated their home dialysis regimen. "It's been like a thousand pounds lifted off my back now that you're off the machine," he told her. She'd repeated her promise that she'd never go on home hemodialysis again.

She'd yet to go through her stack of get-well cards. Her mother and brother, both living on the West Coast, wrote and called often. A number of neighbors and friends also wrote. She wanted to answer all of them, to tell them how well she felt. Carolyn also had a number of pills she had to take every day, and a long list of instructions to remember, most of it concerning self-diagnosis. The key was to be aware of early signs of rejection. The earlier it was caught, the easier it was to stop. The doctors and nurses made her feel her new kidney, its shape and texture. Rejection caused transplanted kidneys to change their shape and soften, and she had to be aware of that. She also carried a small pillow around and often placed it over her lower abdomen to protect the kidney while the incision healed.

That afternoon, Carolyn ventured downstairs to her basement. There in the middle of the rec room was the hemodialysis machine, an ingenious contraption of tubes, filters, and pumps. The "old ball and chain," she called it. It had gathered a thin layer of dust in the three weeks it hadn't been used. Next to it was the bed Carolyn used to lie in during dialysis, and next to that was the easy chair Tom sat in while he monitored the machine. The small black-and-white television set the kids watched had been taken back upstairs. They'd kept it there so the whole family could be together for those three nights a week Carolyn was on the machine.

She heard the front door open and slam shut upstairs, then Greg's footsteps marching around the house.

"Mom," he yelled out.

"I'm downstairs," Carolyn yelled back.

He didn't hear that, and he yelled out "Mom" again, and this time Carolyn detected some anxiety in his voice.

She yelled louder, "I'm in the basement."

He ran downstairs and went immediately to Carolyn and hugged her. She knew from the strength of the hug that when he hadn't seen her upstairs, he'd thought the worst. Although he'd done well in her absence, he'd remained anxious about his mother.

"How'd it go in school?" Carolyn asked.

"Real good. I didn't flunk any tests."

"Did you have any?" she asked.

"Nope," he said.

They both laughed.

Carolyn went over to the corner of the basement where the boxes of unused dialysis filters and unopened cartons of dialysis fluid were stacked.

"Never need them again, right?" Greg asked.

"Those days are gone," Carolyn answered.

In the two years she'd been on home dialysis, she'd never been far from the machine. Although it had kept her alive, it was a symbol of dependence for her.

"Remember the trip to Maine?" Carolyn asked.

"Are you kidding?" Greg answered.

It was two summers ago. The family loved to travel, so they loaded the machine into the trunk of the car and headed for New England. Along the way, Carolyn was dialyzed in the motel room, and once at a campsite in the woods of Maine.

"What are we doing to do with the stuff you won't use?" Greg asked.

"I'm trying to figure that out," Carolyn answered.

Like all kidney patients, Carolyn was the beneficiary of a 1972 federal law that placed kidney disease under Medicare coverage, the only disease so singled out. This was done largely because of public pressures created by wrenching stories of people who'd died either because they couldn't afford dialysis or transplants, or because there were not enough dialysis machines or donor organs available. But now in a climate of medical cost-cutting, questions about the value of spending more than $2 billion a year to keep 60,000 kidney patients alive were arising in and out of government. Published reports alleging Medicare fraud by some of the private dialysis centers that sprang up because of federal reimbursement helped fuel that climate.

Frugality was deeply a part of Carolyn's nature. It had been ingrained in her by her late father, a Los Angeles city fireman who'd managed to save enough to invest in property. Carolyn had always been a saver, a darner of socks, a clipper of coupons. She knew her dialysis machine would be sterilized and reused, but she also thought the filters and fluid could be used by someone else.

That afternoon, Carolyn called her private dialysis center, where she'd gotten the dialysis machine, to tell them she wanted to return the filters and fluid.

"We're really not interested," someone at the center told her.

Carolyn was shocked. "But these are perfectly good. They're still in their original packages," she said.

"It's really not worth it," they said.

"They must be worth hundreds of dollars. Surely somebody could use them," Carolyn argued.

"No, thanks," they said.

This went against her grain. That night over dinner Carolyn complained to Tom. "Just because the government is paying for it, nobody thinks they have to be careful with the money," she said.

"Why don't you see if you can give it to some other kidney organization," he suggested.

The next day, a Friday, she phoned the Kidney Fund in Bethesda, Maryland, a private organization that aided kidney patients. They were happy to receive her gift.

That same day Carolyn was also scheduled to go to the clinic at Walter Reed. Blood tests were run, and she was given a thorough physical examination and found to be in excellent health. Her new kidney functioned perfectly, and there was no indication of rejection.

Betty Landis hauled bags of groceries from the backseat of her Plymouth into the kitchen. For the first time since Matthew's kidney transplant nearly four weeks earlier, they were all eating at home together. Matthew always got better faster at home, so when his condition had stabilized, Dr. McEnery had discharged him.

It was Sunday afternoon and the early April sky was nearly overcast. Small buttons of light peeked through the high clouds. Betty heard the television set blaring from the family room as she put the groceries away. Jim was there with his younger brother Carl, building shelves. Matthew, Valerie, and Janie were watching cartoons. Betty heard Matthew chuckling. The moment he left the hospital, he'd emerged from his shell and become an exuberant little boy again.

Betty heard Jim shouting in the family room, and he sounded anxious. "Matthew!" he yelled. Betty grew uneasy with the tone of Jim's voice and moved toward the doorway that led down to the family room.

"Matthew!" Jim shouted again. At the same moment, Matthew slumped over on the floor. For a split second, Jim thought Matthew was kidding; then he knew he wasn't. It happened that fast.

"My God," Jim cried out. He rushed to Matthew's side and looked down at his ashen face. Matthew's breathing was rapid, shallow, and erratic. Then it stopped, and his eyes rolled back into his head.

"Betty! Betty!" Jim screamed.

She raced over. "Oh, no. What's wrong, what's wrong?"

"It looks like a seizure," he said.

But was it? Jim wondered. Was it a seizure? Heart failure? A brain hemorrhage? Is my son dying right here in front of me?

"Call Children's," he shouted. "Tell them Matthew's unconscious."

Betty ran to the telephone and called the hospital, a number she knew by heart. They had their first lucky break: Dr. McEnery was there.

"Matthew's collapsed," Betty said. "We think he's having a seizure."

McEnery asked for brief details, the look of his eyes, the suddenness of the collapse. Betty told him everything she knew.

"It sounds like a seizure. There's not enough time to get him here. Get him to Mercy South and have them call me immediately. I won't move from this phone."

Betty hung up. She was distraught, and Valerie was off to the side, nearly hysterical. Hold yourself together, Betty told herself. Don't fall apart.

Betty reached for the phone to dial 911 for the rescue squad. Her hands shook too much. Carl raced over to the phone and dialed.

"It's an emergency," he shouted.

Jim gave Matthew mouth-to-mouth resuscitation. Keep oxygen going into him, he kept telling himself, keep the heart, lungs, brain, and kidney going. Keep him alive.

Will the life squad ever get here? Betty wondered. She tried to console Valerie and Janie, and leaned near Jim as he labored over Matthew.

Matthew didn't respond, didn't breathe on his own, didn't show any change at all. He just lay motionless and unconscious. Jim wouldn't quit.

Betty heard the sirens approaching in the distance, such welcome sounds. She opened the door and the paramedics rushed to Matthew. Jim still knelt at his side. The paramedics continued with mouth-to-mouth resuscitation. Matthew remained unconscious.

"We'll take him to Mercy," one of the paramedics said.

They all ran out to the ambulance, Matthew on a stretcher, Jim and Betty following. They leapt into the back of the ambulance. Neighbors had heard the sirens and were out on the street. Carl said he'd stay behind to watch Valerie and Janie.

The ambulance headed for Mercy South Hospital, two miles

away. Jim gripped the side of the truck for balance. He watched Matthew for signs of life as the paramedics continued to work on him. Nothing happened. We're losing him, he thought. After all we've been through, after all he's been through, we're losing him. Betty shared the same thought. They held hands as the sirens howled and the ambulance raced.

"Do you know what might have caused the seizure?" a paramedic asked.

Jim wasn't sure. He thought it might be the drug Matthew was taking to fight off rejection. He had been released from Children's two days earlier. On Saturday and Sunday mornings Jim had driven Matthew back there for injections of the potent steroid Solu-Medrol. Both times the doctors warned Jim that seizures were a possible side effect. But Matthew had taken it before without any problem. Why would he have a seizure this time? Jim had no answer, only an unshakable dread.

The ambulance slowed as it rounded a corner and turned into the hospital emergency room entrance. Jim and Betty still saw no signs of life in Matthew.

They both feared that physicians without full knowledge of Matthew's medical history would be on very uncertain ground.

"Call Dr. McEnery at Children's Hospital," Jim told a doctor. "My son has just had a kidney transplant."

The Mercy South doctor called McEnery immediately. Matthew is having a seizure, he told him. It was a quandary for McEnery. If Matthew remained in his seizure, it could cost him his life. But if they used the drugs they normally use to combat seizures, phenobarbital or Dilantin, they would block the effects of the immune-suppression drugs. This could lead to an equally precarious problem: the rejection of Matthew's kidney. McEnery thought quickly. There was one possible solution: Valium. It might bring him out of his seizure, and it wouldn't block the immune-suppression drugs.

The physicians at Mercy South put an intravenous line into

Matthew and began the Valium. They told Jim and Betty that Matthew needed to be rushed to Children's.

The ambulance driver said only one of Matthew's parents could ride.

"You go," Jim said to Betty. "Carl and I will follow you."

The ambulance sped toward Children's Hospital. A paramedic steadied the Valium solution dripping into Matthew's right arm. He'd started to breathe on his own again. A good sign. An oxygen mask covered his small face. Betty watched him and thought, Will he be brain-damaged? Will he lose his kidney? Will he lose his life? Matthew remained unconscious.

A volunteer fireman drove Jim home. He and Carl loaded the two girls in the car, dropped them off at Jim's parents' house, explained what was going on very briefly, and raced toward Children's, twenty minutes behind the ambulance.

Dr. McEnery was waiting at the emergency room door when the ambulance arrived. He'd seen some children go into seizures like this and not come out of them. The ambulance doors opened. Matthew's eyes stayed rolled back in his head.

"Get him right in here," someone yelled.

Matthew's stretcher was wheeled into the ER. McEnery probed and touched him; there was no response. The Valium kept dripping. When was he going to come out of this? Would he come out of this? McEnery was calm and methodical, and worried.

Betty studied Matthew for any movement or twitching, anything that would tell her he was coming to. There was none. Matthew remained on oxygen, under the bright overhead lights of the ER, as the doctors checked and rechecked, looking for change.

Jim arrived, out of breath. "How's he doing?"

"There's no change," Betty told him.

They kept watching. Minutes took hours to pass. McEnery and a small cluster of doctors and nurses stood over Matthew, talking, probing, hoping he'd react. By chance, Betty and Jim met their church pastor. He sat and talked with Betty, and they knelt and prayed together on a bench just outside the emergency room.

At least thirty minutes had passed since Matthew had arrived at Children's, more than an hour since his seizure.

Then Betty and Jim heard it at the same time. It was a low, groaning cry. "Mommmm . . ." It was Matthew's voice. He was coming to. "Mommm . . ." he repeated.

"I'm right here Matthew, I'm right here. . . . I'm not going to leave you," Betty repeated, standing at his side.

Matthew stirred and slowly recognized Jim and Betty looking down at him. "You're going to be fine, Matthew," Jim assured him. Jim gripped Betty's hand and they held on to one another.

The doctors kept examining Matthew. "Follow my finger with your eyes, Matthew," one said. He moved his finger to the right, Matthew's eyes moved to the right with it. Then to the left, and Matthew's eyes followed again.

"Very good, Matthew, very good." It was a very positive sign. They tested his reflexes. They were normal. There appeared to be no serious neurological damage. His brain and body were intact.

With relief in his voice, McEnery told Jim and Betty, "It looks like he's doing pretty well. He's come out of this in good shape."

They stayed at Matthew's side, assuring him he wasn't alone. Groggy from his seizure and the Valium, he said nothing.

McEnery had no explanation why Solu-Medrol had suddenly caused a seizure now in Matthew when it hadn't in the past. "I think we need to run him through some more neurological tests just to make sure he's doing as well as we think he is," McEnery told Jim. "I think it's wise to hold him here at least overnight."

Jim and Betty agreed.

"Neurology will have to run some tests to rule some things out," McEnery said. "I don't think there's much more for me to do around here."

"Thanks for being here when we needed you," Jim said.

"It comes with the territory," McEnery said as he turned to leave.

Although McEnery and the other physicians strongly suspected that Solu-Medrol was the cause of Matthew's seizure, they were not completely certain. They were concerned about infections and they needed to rule them out, as well as other potential causes.

Matthew needed to be protected from possible infections, and a young woman doctor, a resident newly assigned to the kidney unit, ordered Matthew to the isolation unit on Three South. Within the past few days, Matthew had developed blisters that Jim and Betty knew tests had shown were caused by a self-limiting form of herpes called herpes simplex. Now as Matthew was taken up in the elevator and wheeled down a long corridor toward the isolation unit, they were stunned to learn the doctor was planning to put Matthew in the isolation unit with a boy who had chicken pox. Chicken pox is also caused by a herpes virus, but a different type from Matthew's. These viruses do not have cross-immunities, meaning that Matthew would be vulnerable to chicken pox, which was a far more dangerous form of herpes for him. Chicken pox is also one of the most contagious of all diseases.

"You can't put Matthew in with someone who has chicken pox," Jim told the doctor.

Taken aback, the doctor answered firmly, "There is no problem. They have the same type of herpes." Her logic was simple. If they had the same type of herpes, then Matthew was being exposed to something he already had, and there was no danger.

Jim knew better. He could feel his muscles tighten. "They don't have the same type of herpes, that's my point. Matthew has herpes simplex. I know because I had it myself once. This other boy has chicken pox, and I know that's not herpes simplex. You can't expose him to that boy."

The young doctor was insistent. So was Jim. "Why don't you go check your own records if you won't take my word for it? They did a culture on Matthew earlier in the week," he told her.

Jim was encouraged that she took the time to check, but when she came back a few minutes later she told Jim and Betty there was no record of the culture. It apparently had been taken before the end of the month, and now, at the beginning of the new month, there was a changeover of personnel and it could not be located.

"I'm positive Matthew has simplex," Jim repeated.

"If it were simplex he wouldn't have blisters on his side," the doctor answered.

Jim was starting to lose his self-control.

"Goddammit," he shouted, "I know the blisters are unusual, but I'm telling you it's still herpes simplex."

Nothing he said seemed to impress her. She was going by the book. She asked another young doctor to examine Matthew, and he agreed with her. She wouldn't listen to Jim, and her voice had a strong hint of annoyance.

An orderly pushed Matthew's stretcher toward the isolation room. Jim blocked the doorway with his body. There was an air of unreality about the situation. He couldn't believe what was happening. Betty stood off to the side, supporting Jim, but uncomfortable about confronting hospital authority.

The doctor's tone turned sharp. "Mr. Landis . . . please."

Jim glared at her. He didn't budge. Betty hoped something would happen to end the impasse.

"I'm not going to move, dammit. He has herpes simplex. I've told you that, and I don't know what else I can do to convince you."

She moved the stretcher toward the isolation unit again, and Jim grabbed it and didn't let go.

"Could you please check with the other doctors who've taken care of Matthew?" he asked.

"I already have, Mr. Landis. They agree with me. Now will you please move out of the way," she said. Jim didn't know if she was telling the truth, but he realized she would not relent.

He tried to sort things out in his mind. One moment he considered pulling the stretcher away and taking Matthew to another hospital. He realized quickly that was ridiculous, and risky to Matthew. Above all, he didn't want to jeopardize Matthew. His knuckles were white from gripping the stretcher's metal bars, and he felt a bit foolish standing there. He looked down at Matthew, who was groggy and half asleep and not aware of the battle going on around him. He tried to weigh the potential harm to his son. He looked at the doctor, then at Matthew. "You win," he said, releasing his grip.

The doctor said nothing as the stretcher moved into the isolation unit. Matthew was placed just a few feet from the boy with chicken pox. They were the only two in the unit.

Jim and Betty stood side by side outside of the isolation unit, watching through the glass as the orderlies and nurses lifted Matthew onto the bed. Jim turned to Betty and said, "If they're wrong, I'm gonna burn their ass." Betty had never seen him so angry.

"It's the arrogance I can't stand," he said. "She acted as if we didn't know a damn thing."

"I'm scared," Betty said.

Jim was scared too. They walked to a bench in the hallway and sat down. It had been the most emotionally exhausting day of their lives. The fatigue drained their spirit. Jim rested his head in his hands and turned to Betty. "Why don't you go home and get some sleep? I'm gonna stay here the night and have this looked into in the morning."

"You sure you're all right?" Betty asked.

"I'll be okay. It's just that I can't quite believe all this yet."

They could see the weariness in each other's eyes. They walked to the vending machines for a sandwich and coffee and sat at a table in the cafeteria. They were alone. They heard the monotonous hum of the floor waxer as it slithered down the corridor. They both hoped they were wrong about the herpes, but they didn't think so. They kissed goodbye and embraced for several moments, as if shielding one another from harm.

Betty drove home at about eight, numbed of all feeling. She just wanted to put her arms around Valerie and Janie. Jim walked to the visitors area to sleep on a sofa. He found little rest that night.

When there was a problem on the kidney unit at Children's Hospital, the call went out for the "white hair." That was Dr. Clark West, a tall, slender man in his midsixties who was one of the founding fathers of pediatric kidney care in this country and chief of the kidney division at Children's. He had a controlled, almost distant, manner, a penetrating mind, and a full head of white hair.

Jim and Betty had known Dr. West for three years and for much of that time felt uneasy in his presence. He always looked at the floor or the ceiling when he talked to them, and never expressed any emotion. He just calmly recited the facts, and for a long time they thought he was unfeeling. But soon after Matthew's second transplant, when his rejection was so acute it brought him near death, Clark West had walked into Matthew's hospital room alone one afternoon. Jim and Betty watched silently from the corner. West did not see them. He stood at the foot of the bed in a dim light and stared at Matthew, not saying a word. He then turned and walked out. As he turned, Jim had seen West's eyes, and that day learned what everyone at Children's knew: beneath Dr. West's aloofness was a man deeply vulnerable to the suffering of his young patients.

Clark West seldom made rounds or visited patients' rooms anymore. Because of Matthew, this Monday morning was an exception. Betty had driven to the hospital early in the morning, and she and Jim were already in Matthew's isolation room, masked and gowned. Dr. West came in followed by a small group of physicians. The small, pale-green room grew crowded. He nodded hello to Jim and Betty and went quickly to Matthew's side. He pulled back the blanket and reached in to touch one of Matthew's blisters. Matthew didn't react in any way. Blisters from the chicken pox virus are painful, herpes simplex blisters are not.

Dr. West glanced up with a hard look in his eye. "Move this boy out of this room!" He didn't have to say immediately. Jim had been right. Within seconds, Matthew was removed from the isolation room.

Betty shuddered. My God, what now? She looked at Jim. She saw his worried eyes over the sterile mask. He shook his head. They strained to hear as the doctors spoke to one another. They picked up a word here, an expression there, confirming their worst fears. Betty grew frustrated. Why hadn't the doctor known enough to touch Matthew's blisters the night before?

Outside the isolation unit, Dr. West admitted the mistake and Jim grew angry all over again. Yes, the hospital had saved his son's life more than once, but this was close to inexcusable. And it wasn't just that they'd made a mistake, but also the fact that he had told the doctor it was wrong and she'd refused to listen. Dr. West said he understood their feelings and that the doctors would do all they could. Jim then went to the hospital's patient representative, a kind of ombudsman, and registered a formal complaint about the episode that was circulated to a number of department heads at the hospital. The ombudsman was courteous and helpful, and Jim told him that if anything happened to Matthew because of this, he would sue the hospital. The representative said he understood.

In Matthew's room a little while later, the young woman resident who had put Matthew in isolation the night before quietly approached Jim and Betty. She was exceedingly solicitous and asked if there was anything she could do. Jim and Betty were incredulous. She still could not bring herself to apologize. They reacted to her very coolly, and she left the room.

Clark West was worried. He'd long admired the fight and spirit in Matthew. He'd hoped for three years that he and his colleagues could put together the right blend of science, art, and luck to give Matthew a good kidney and a long life. To think they themselves might have jeopardized all that was almost intolerable to him. He called a meeting of experts in his office. "We've got a problem," he announced.

Dr. McEnery was there, as was an infectious-diseases expert from the University of Cincinnati School of Medicine, a neurologist, and Dr. Frederic Strife, a member of the kidney team. They all realized the situation was perilous. "I feel like we're walking along the edge of a diving board, blindfolded," one of the doctors said.

They sat in a small circle in West's comfortable office, their expressions grim. They reasoned from every angle and tried to squeeze every drop of information from every test and every symptom they knew about. Dr. West was certain that Matthew's infection was herpes simplex. The infectious-diseases expert agreed. They all had to face up to the fact that Matthew had been exposed to chicken pox for fifteen hours. Dr. West was not in a mood to blame anyone now. What can we do to correct it? he asked.

They looked at lab reports that showed that Matthew's kidney-function numbers had worsened. What was the cause? Was it an infection, or another rejection episode? The numbers didn't tell you. Was the chicken pox virus already invading Matthew's cells? Should they withdraw all the immune-suppression drugs now so he could fight that infection?

Paul McEnery sifted all the options and then spoke. "If we take him off the immune suppressants, what are we really telling Matthew and his family? I think we're saying, 'We can't save your kidney, and there's a good chance your life won't be very long.' It's likely to be the beginning of the end for him." Everyone knew McEnery was right.

They examined another option, zoster-immune globulin. The chicken pox virus is in the herpes zoster viral family, and this experimental globulin, if given to Matthew within the next several hours, could establish antibodies against chicken pox. Cincinnati Children's didn't have the globulin. They immediately called Children's Hospital in Boston. It was put on the next plane to Cincinnati.

Questions still hung in the air. Would the globulin work? Or would the chicken pox still take hold? If he did get the chicken pox, the consequences to Matthew with his compromised immunity could be devastating. Their best guess was that Matthew's worsening numbers were caused by another rejection episode, not infection. With the globulin on its way from Boston, and continued use of immune-suppression drugs, they might be able to prevent the chicken pox, save Matthew, and also save his kidney. "A triple play," one doctor hopefully called it.

To accomplish all this was a calculated gamble based on their experience, judgment, and intuition. If they proved right, Matthew and his parents would escape with nothing more than a bad scare; if they were wrong, everything could be lost.

The meeting in Dr. West's office broke up, and the doctors met with Jim and Betty in a small conference room. They laid out their diagnosis and plan of action.

116

"We think the numbers are getting worse because of another rejection," Dr. West said. "We don't want to cut back the immune suppression."

"What if he gets chicken pox?" Jim asked.

"We think the globulin should take care of that. If it doesn't, we'll have to stop the drugs . . ." West said.

"And that means he'll lose this kidney," Jim said.

Their silence was all the answer Jim needed.

Betty studied their expressions. They all seemed so grim, she thought. It didn't inspire optimism.

Jim asked the hard question. "How could something like this have happened?"

"We're not perfect," McEnery said. "It was just a terrible mistake."

Jim knew they felt bad, perhaps even guilty. But this was small consolation. He wanted to know what was next.

"How long will it be before we have some answers?" he asked.

"We'll be watching him closely for at least seventy-two hours," McEnery said. "We should know where we stand then."

"Is the globulin getting here soon?" Jim wanted to know.

"It's coming in tonight, and as soon as we get it, we're giving it to him," West said.

Jim and Betty thanked them for meeting with them, and they all wished one another good luck.

Jim and Betty walked down the corridor back to Matthew's room. They entered, masked and smiling, to allay Matthew's fears.

Betty had brought Curious George from home that morning and had given him to Matthew, who cradled George next to him.

"How's George feeling?" Betty asked.

Matthew had grown silent again, but his eyes remained fiercely alert. He turned to George and whispered, then looked up at his parents.

117

"George is sick again," he said.

Jim and Betty could see in Matthew's eyes that he was not well.

"You tell George that he's going to get well real soon, and so are you," Jim said.

Matthew studied Jim's eyes and again turned to George, but said nothing more.

Jim couldn't remember a more exhausting thirty-hour period in his life. He'd been through the gamut of emotions from fear, to rage, to anxiety, back to fear, and now, to a small fragment of hope. He'd lost all sense of time, but he knew it was growing dark outside so it must be late afternoon. He'd already called work to tell them he couldn't be in tonight. He told Betty and Matthew he was going for a little walk and left the room. He went to the chapel on the first floor.

More than a year ago, around Christmastime, Jim had come to this chapel when Matthew was ill after the rejection of his second kidney. Matthew's weight had fallen to nearly his birth weight, and he had infections and a perforated bowel, was punctured with needles, and couldn't keep any food down. Jim was at his low point and thought it cruel to keep Matthew going. He prayed that if God was going to take him, to please take him soon and end his son's suffering and pain. But Matthew rallied, surprising everyone, and Jim never repeated that prayer. Now Jim knelt down before the small altar, bowed his head, and prayed quietly. "Dear Lord, please don't let my son die."

~~~~~~~~~~ S E V E N

Jo Leslie stood at the front of a large conference room and ignored the small lectern so she could have a more direct conversation with her audience. It was a Tuesday morning and she was spreading the word about organ donation. This was how Jo spent her time when she wasn't directly procuring human organs. Getting the message out was crucial because the need for organs was so great.

Five to ten thousand people were waiting for kidneys around the country, and Jo realized probably less than half would get a kidney transplant this year. Others awaited livers, pancreases, corneas, and hearts. There were a number of reasons for this shortage. Of those who died in hospitals, only one percent died under conditions that permitted organ donation, in short, brain death. Of that number, many families were not even approached about organ donation. Despite its growing success in the 1980s, the idea of organ transplantation still had not reached down into the bedrock of medicine. It wasn't taught in medical schools, and many medical professionals away from major hospitals regarded it as outside medicine's mainstream. Because of this, doctors often were reluctant to get involved. One doctor had even prevented Jo from talking to a potential donor family. "It would be too much for them," he'd told Jo.

Some doctors feared families might sue them if they declared a family member brain dead and opened the door to donation.

Some didn't want to expend the extra effort organ donation required, and others simply were ignorant. Whatever the reasons, Jo sought to break down the barriers that prevented potential organs from getting to the people who needed them, for the sake of the recipients and potential donor families.

She faced other obstacles that frustrated her and her attempts to procure more kidneys. The hardest was when kidneys were donated but not used. Sometimes they weren't used because the surgeon removing them did not cut them out properly, so they could not be transplanted. Sometimes donor blood types made matches difficult. This was especially true of AB blood types. Kidneys from AB donors could only go to AB recipients, and they are very rare.

But the major reason human organs were discarded was because they ran out of time. They would go to a transplant center but fail to pass the cross-match test, which determined whether the donor organ was compatible with the recipient. The organs then went to the next center, and maybe the one after that, in search of a suitable recipient. Each stop took at least eight to ten hours, until forty-eight or more hours were gone, and the organs became unusable.

Nationally, 25 percent of all donor kidneys had to be discarded. One of Jo's proudest accomplishments was cutting down the kidney-discard rate in her center to about half the national rate, and half of what it was before she arrived.

But she still had failures. Recently, the glue that held parts of one of their perfusion machines together had seeped into the perfusion fluid. Two kidneys were destroyed. She'd felt like kicking the machine.

In some respects, organ procurement was like a ministry. You needed human sensitivity to help people in great distress, and you had to proselytize your faith in organ donation wherever people would listen. Jo took her message to many places. Recently she'd spoken before the Rotary Club, and a few weeks earlier she'd spoken to a church group. It had taken the congregation a few minutes to realize she wasn't there to talk about donations for the new church organ. Today she spoke to twenty neurologic nurses from a number of Baltimore area hospitals.

"There is nothing you can do to diminish the pain a family feels when they've suddenly lost someone they love," she told them. "You can't bring that person back for them, but you can do something to help these families, and that's organ donation. It is an opportunity to have something good come out of a senseless tragedy, and it may help lessen the absurdity and futility of the loss these families feel. You can be a part of that."

Jo wore a white lab coat and gestured with her hands. The nurses, sitting in rows of desks in a third-floor room at University Hospital in Baltimore, listened intently. "The accidents that can result in organ donation usually happen late at night; often it's a head injury to someone who's young. Maybe you've been on duty eight or ten hours already and you're tired. I understand that. I realize the last thing you want to do is get involved with organ donation, because you know it's going to take more time and you just want to get out of the place and go home. I want to impress on you that you should stay, and you should consider organ donation, not because it's easy, but because it is important and because it's the right thing to do. It's why you're in medicine!"

Because her organ-procurement center coordinated organ donation and distribution around the state of Maryland, Jo delivered her message as far west as Cumberland and all the way over to the Eastern Shore and the Chesapeake Bay. She spoke to doctors and nurses who worked in intensive care units, emergency rooms, operating rooms, and other parts of the hospitals where they could help families give a final gift so that others could live on. She wanted to establish a statewide network that would produce more usable organs, and to do it she had to gain the trust, confidence, and understanding of these people.

Jo wound up her talk by discussing some of the technical details of managing patients who are potential organ donors, and a question and answer session followed. A young nurse raised her hand and asked who should approach the donor family first.

"In most cases, I or a member of my staff will," Jo answered, "but it is also helpful if you or a doctor also speak to them before we arrive."

A second nurse asked, "If a patient has an organ-donation card, does that mean we can legally take organs if he or she is pronounced brain dead?"

"Even with that card we will not take organs unless we have the permission of the next of kin," Jo explained. "They must always be asked and their wishes must always be honored. The family has to live on, and we don't want to make that death any harder on them than it already is."

"How can you explain brain death to lay people?" another nurse asked.

"I don't. I just tell the family that it's the end and there is nothing that can be done. You don't want them lingering with false hope."

A young nurse asked a personal question. "We all deal with death in our work, but you have to face it all the time. How can you stand it?"

Jo paused for a second and spoke slowly. "I'd be lying if I said it wasn't hard. Life matters to me a lot and it disturbs me terribly when I see someone who isn't going to have enough of it. Talking to the donor families isn't easy. I think we all want to turn away from people who've suffered a shock like that. But you have to feel you're making a difference in their lives, that you're serving an important function that can help them deal with grief. That may sound cut and dried, but it's how I have to approach it, and it's how I hope you would approach it."

The questions came to an end. Jo told the nurses she appreciated their attention, and several broke into light applause.

Jo took the elevator to her sixth-floor office. She hung up her lab coat on a hanger near the door and walked to her desk. She leaned back in her chair and took a sip of coffee and looked over her statistics. Her office was supposed to procure sixty-three organs for the year. As of now, they had already placed thirty-seven with eight months to go. That gratified her, but she didn't base her success only on numbers. Increasingly she felt a debt to the donor families, and she wanted them to feel a strong sense of purpose in what they did. That meant taking extra care and time, and time was always at a premium.

She examined the red splotches on her arm. To her they were unsightly, like some ugly skin disease. She assumed they were caused by an allergy to the perfusion fluid, because she'd never had them before she worked in organ procurement.

Jo glanced at her schedule. Tomorrow she had an organ-procurement training program in Salisbury, Maryland, that would take most of the day. Salisbury was a long drive, but it was a large hospital with potential for donor organs. On Thursday she was scheduled to talk to nurses at Union Memorial Hospital in Baltimore.

She hit the rewind button on her phone answering machine and played the messages back. One was from Karin Earp, the transplant coordinator at The Johns Hopkins Hospital, confirming their lunch date. Jo reset the machine to answer incoming calls and left for lunch.

The nighttime air of early April was cool and dry, and Louise Kelly peeked through her kitchen window to see the fading light of the evening sky. Her husband, Eugene, was in the backyard, digging up the vegetable garden with a pitchfork. She put the last of the dinner dishes in the cupboard and heard a joyful scream from upstairs. It was Elizabeth, the seven-year-old foster child the Kellys had taken in three months earlier. She always hollered when she took her nightly bath. Foster children had been a part of the Kellys' family for years. They'd now taken in more than thirty of them. It seemed natural to Louise. She'd grown up in a working-class neighborhood in Trenton, New Jersey, and her mother took in neighborhood children when their parents had trouble. As a young girl, Louise had gotten up many mornings and nearly tripped over a sleeping child, taken in by her mother late the night before. Caring for children was something Louise did because they were special creatures, "little miracles" she called them, and they all needed love and attention.

The front door popped open. "It's me," Maureen announced.

Maureen walked to the kitchen and Louise turned to her and smiled. Maureen hid the sense of shock and sadness that struck her when she saw her mother's drawn, tired face. She knew she hadn't been sleeping well since the accident.

"Want a cup of coffee?" Louise asked.

"Love one," Maureen answered.

Maureen took her cup into the living room. Lisa's picture was still displayed on the fireplace mantel. On an end table was a framed letter Maureen had written to her parents. She'd given it to them one recent Christmas and in it she expressed her love for them. "My wish is that my children grow up to love and respect me, as much as I do you," she'd said. Louise and Eugene treasured the letter.

Eugene came in from outside. He smiled and said hello to Maureen and went to the bathroom to wash his hands. He settled into his favorite easy chair near the foot of the stairs, and the two foster children, Elizabeth and Jason, who was five, crept down and crawled into his lap. Both were bathed and dressed in their pajamas. They snuggled next to Eugene as he opened his arms to them.

Louise returned from the kitchen and sat across from Maureen. Maureen had visited her parents more often since Lisa's death and spoke to her mother at least once a day on the phone.

Elizabeth and Jason stayed on Eugene's lap as eight o'clock drew near. "Getting to be bedtime," he told them.

They untangled themselves slowly. "Can't we stay up . . . please?" Elizabeth pleaded.

"No, young lady. You have to get your rest," Louise said.

The children gave Louise and Eugene a hug and a wet kiss and scampered upstairs, lingering for a moment near the top until Louise told them once more to get to bed. Already upstairs was Debbie, a pretty nine-year-old foster child who had lived with the Kellys for several years. They were in the process of legally adopting her, a decision made long before Lisa's death. Safely out of earshot, Louise said, "Those two will stay up all night if you let them." Both had come from bad home situations and it had taken a long time for them to become trusting and open.

Maureen took a sip of coffee. "How's Ellen doing?" she asked.

Louise shrugged her shoulders. "I wish I knew. She's so quiet. I know a lot is going on inside, but she doesn't let on a thing. I mentioned counseling to her and she snapped at me. 'Do you think I'm crazy?' she said. I said, 'Of course not,' and she walked away, like she didn't want to listen."

"You know she's hurting," Maureen said.

"A lot, an awful lot," Louise said. "Sometimes I think she doesn't talk about it because she doesn't want to hurt me, then sometimes I think she just doesn't want to talk about it."

Ellen was not the only family member to withdraw. The Kellys' older natural son, Donald, who'd fled Shocktrauma the second he heard how badly Lisa was hurt, still would not utter her name. He'd attended her funeral, but he walked out of the room if her name came up in conversation. He did not visit the cemetery where she was buried.

They heard the click of a heel on a wooden step coming from the top of the stairs. It was Ellen. She walked down slowly, wearing a plaid blouse and blue jeans. Her dark hair was neatly combed and her complexion was clear and clean, but her eyes had a distant look to them.

"Hi, hon," Maureen said. "How you doin'?"

Ellen looked at Maureen and smiled. "Okay, I guess," she said. She walked through the living room to the kitchen, where she sliced herself a piece of cake and took it back up to her bedroom. "Goodnight," she said as she passed through.

Louise shook her head again. "That's all you ever get out of her, one or two words at a time."

Eugene Kelly sipped his coffee. He'd said little and appeared restless. "You've been kind of quiet, Dad," Maureen said.

"Yeah," he said, stroking his chin, "been thinking about that telephone call again."

Maureen wasn't sure what he was talking about, but her mother's look told her not to ask.

Eugene Kelly began to unravel a strange story. In December, three months before Lisa's accident, he had been unable to sleep one night and was up at 2 A.M. watching television when the telephone rang. A call at that time of night is always unnerving, and when he answered it he heard the voice of a young woman, perhaps a girl. She did not identify herself and he didn't recognize her voice. She asked if he had a daughter named Lisa. "Yes, I do," he answered. "She's been in a car accident," the voice said, "and she's been taken to Shocktrauma in Baltimore."

"That's impossible," he answered. "She's right upstairs in bed." Nonetheless, he raced upstairs, grabbed a flashlight, and ran inside Lisa's room and shined it into her eyes. She awoke. "What do you want?" she asked, startled.

"Nothing, honey, just go back to sleep. I'm sorry I woke you."

He returned downstairs to tell the caller she was mistaken, but when he picked up the phone no one was on the line.

126

"Maybe it was a dream," Maureen said.

Eugene paused for a second. "It wasn't a dream. I don't dream things like that."

They knew better than to push it. Eugene Kelly was not one to mistake a dream for reality. He didn't pursue it any more and seemed content to drop it. So did Maureen and her mother.

It was now past nine and Maureen prepared to leave.

"Did I ever show you the letter from Jo Leslie?" Louise asked. "It came a few days ago."

"No, you didn't."

Louise went to a drawer and pulled out the neatly folded letter. Maureen read it over. It told briefly of the four people who had received Lisa's organs, and of the research made possible by their donation.

Maureen wept as she read it. "It gives you hope that at least something good may come out of it," she said.

Louise spoke. "You wonder about those people. You can't help it. I wonder what they're like, how they're doing."

"It makes sense that one of her kidneys went to a young child, doesn't it?" Maureen said.

Louise nodded. "He's the one I think about most."

The small color television set in the corner of Matthew's hospital room was on, but he paid it little attention. He'd drawn deeper into himself since his exposure to the chicken pox virus. He seldom spoke, seldom acknowledged anything. His eyes followed everyone and studied all their expressions, but he showed little emotion himself. He clung tightly to Curious George while his anxious parents and doctors all awaited the answer to the question that still hung heavily: Was this third kidney transplant the charm, or the final strike? Matthew seemed to be waiting for the same answer.

He was constantly probed and poked, studied like a specimen under a microscope. Blood was drawn, his temperature taken, cultures examined. A computerized axial tomography (CAT) scan revealed no neurological problem, meaning his seizure was almost certainly caused by the drug Solu-Medrol. That was good news. But his kidney-function numbers remained poor, and he was listless and pale. He'd also had a second, milder seizure. Only time would reveal if he had a systemic viral infection, or was in a worsening state of rejection, or would escape this very risky period unharmed. The more time that passed without signs of infection, the better his prospects. Forty-eight hours had gone by since his exposure to chicken pox. Another twenty-four to forty-eight hours were needed.

Jim and Betty talked with the doctors several times each day to pick up any scrap of information. The doctors were always friendly, and evasive. "We just don't know yet," they'd say. "We should know more tomorrow." Each tomorrow was just as uncertain.

Matthew had a slight lisp and had never been able to say his name quite right. It came out "Matu." It became a nickname, as did "Bubby," a version of brother. Every day during their wait, Jim and Betty called Matthew these pet names, trying to coax a smile out of him. Matthew just stared and said nothing. At night when Jim hugged him goodbye, Matthew's return hug felt weak. It went this way for more than three anxious days.

On Friday morning, Jim walked into Matthew's room about 8 A.M., and Matthew greeted him with a smile. It lighted the room more than the sunlight beaming in through the windows. Matthew's cheeks were pink, his fever gone, his spirit back. Joy and relief swept over Jim. He forgot his fatigue and sought out Dr. McEnery.

McEnery was smiling. "His numbers are looking very good," he said. "He shows no sign of an infection and the rejection episode seems to be over. I think we're over the hump."

Jim rushed to a pay phone to call Betty. "Looks like we got

our little boy back," he told her. They laughed and cried at the same time.

"Dad? Can I paint?" Matthew asked when Jim returned.

Jim set up his paper and paints, and Matthew paused.

"I paint truck," Matthew said. He painted a fleet of them, all red.

Later, Matthew ate lunch with a flourish and returned to painting. Then he watched cartoons on television, and especially enjoyed Tom and Jerry. By midafternoon it was time for Jim to leave.

"I've got to be off to work, Matthew. Mom'll be here in a little while," Jim said.

Matthew understood. Jim leaned over Matthew's bed and reached out to hug him, and Matthew wrapped his arms around Jim's neck. Jim felt his son's tiny arms squeezing him hard. "Careful, Bubby," he kidded, "you're so strong you're about to squeeze my head off."

Jim broke into a broad grin as he looked down at his son; he was smiling and giggling.

Linda Blanchard wanted to know how her mother felt about having someone else's kidney in her body. At fifteen, Linda was curious about many things, but the fact that she knew her mother's kidney donor was a young girl close to her own age heightened her interest.

It was early evening and she and her mother were in their station wagon, headed along Rockville Pike to the Congressional Shopping Plaza in the Washington suburbs.

"Do you think about the girl who gave you her kidney?" Linda asked.

"I think about her often," Carolyn answered.

Linda was still curious. "What kind of things do you think about when you think of her?"

"I don't really picture a person in my mind. It's more of a sense than anything else. I told your dad, it's like a bond with a relative or an old friend you haven't seen in a long time."

"If something like that happened to me, would you donate my organs?" Linda asked.

The question chilled Carolyn. "Of course I would," she said, but it was clear she didn't want to talk about it, and Linda let it drop.

Linda's curiosity appeared to be satisfied. Carolyn had few worries about her daughter. She worried more about Greg. She thought he was the family member who most benefited from her organ transplant. She'd realized her illness had pained him deeply, even though he seldom said so directly. A few days after Carolyn had gotten out of the hospital, he'd hugged her and said, "I'm real grateful to that girl's family." That's how Carolyn felt, too.

The next morning, a Friday, Carolyn went to Walter Reed for her routine checkup. It was about a forty-minute trip and she'd made it twice a week since her transplant more than a month earlier. She hoped it would soon be cut back to once a week because she'd been doing so well.

Carolyn's main contact there was Kathy Oddenino, the transplant nurse whom Carolyn had known since she first came to Walter Reed five years earlier. Kathy had long experience with organ-transplant patients. Divorced and the mother of six grown children, she dealt with the problems her patients brought, some physical, many emotional.

Her office was in the fourth-floor kidney unit. She'd decorated it with prints and a red wall poster that read: NOBODY LOVES LIFE LIKE A NURSE. Carolyn sat across from Kathy's desk.

"Your numbers look very good, Carolyn," Kathy said. "So does your hematocrit." Carolyn's hematocrit level, a measure of her red-blood-cell count, had gone from a third of normal into the normal range. Red blood cells carry oxygen, and when they're diminished, a result of disease and hemodialysis, energy levels drop, one reason Carolyn had been so fatigued on dialysis.

Kathy looked over Carolyn's X rays. Her heart had returned to normal size. It had enlarged considerably while she was on hemodialysis. In virtually every way, her body was returning to normal.

"Everything about you seems healthy," Kathy said. "Now let me look you over."

Kathy and Carolyn moved down the hall to a small examining room where Kathy took Carolyn's blood pressure. It was 140 over 85, a little high but within the normal range.

"Have you had symptoms of any kind?" Kathy asked.

"None, I've felt wonderful."

Kathy put a stethoscope to Carolyn's chest and listened. Her lungs were clear; her heartbeat even and strong. Her temperature was normal. Then Kathy palpated the incision and the outline of the kidney.

"The kidney feels very good," Kathy said.

She asked Carolyn about each of her pills and their purposes. Carolyn knew some of them, such as Imuran and Prednisone, were for rejection, but she was uncertain about the purpose of some of the others. Kathy emphasized to her that she had to know everything about each drug she took.

"I have them all written down on a list that I keep in the kitchen," Carolyn explained.

"I know, but I want you to memorize them," Kathy said. "If you're ever seen by another doctor, you're going to know a lot more about all of this than he will. You've got to be able to explain everything, especially with your plans to move to the West Coast in a few months."

Carolyn said she understood and promised she'd have them all memorized next time.

"How are things at home?" Kathy asked.

"They're going very well. The children are doing well and Tom's gearing up to leave the army."

"How's he feel about being passed over?"

"I think he's over his disappointment."

Kathy knew how much Carolyn's family meant to her. She also knew from experience that many retired military officers feel lost and unattached after leaving the service. She was concerned Tom might develop problems that could add more stress to Carolyn's life.

Carolyn left the examining room and spoke briefly to two young sisters she knew. The older sister had suffered a rare

132

blood disease that destroyed her kidneys, and she had received a kidney from her younger sister.

"How are you girls doing?" Carolyn asked.

"Great. You look good too," said Sharon, the older sister.

"I'm feeling so good I can't believe it," Carolyn answered. "I didn't think I'd ever have this much energy."

"I feel the same way," Sharon said. "The difference is incredible."

Carolyn took the elevator to the first-floor lobby, a large, cavernous room with military and medical personnel moving in and out. It was midday and the sun was warm. She had a number of errands ahead of her, buying groceries, picking up some yarn for knitting, and cooking dinner. For the first time in five years, the thought of those tasks didn't overwhelm her. She felt like a whole person again.

It was a lazy Baltimore Sunday. Jo sat in the family room of a friend's home, one of a small gathering, enjoying brunch. Sunlight poured through the windows, and she could see the buds on the tree branches outside. They talked, sipped coffee, munched on rolls, bagels, and scrambled eggs.

"What do you do?" a woman she'd just met asked her.

"I work in organ procurement," Jo answered.

Nancy, the hostess and a close friend of Jo's, overheard. She thought Jo's work was almost heroic, but she also thought she sometimes detected a sadness in Jo. She looked over at Jo. "Tell her what you *really* do."

Jo smiled politely. She told the woman that she talked with families to ask if they would consider donating the organs of their family member and, if they agreed, tried to place those organs. She told of a case that past Friday night when she went to Shocktrauma and spoke with the family of an accident victim. Jo's description was sparse, devoid of feeling. It was just a job, she said. The woman, who appeared to be about Jo's age, asked Jo if she saw the results of what she did. Jo answered, "You don't usually see them, but you know they're there. We talk to other organ-procurement coordinators in other areas, so we learn about many of the people for whom we've gotten organs. It's not always a success story, but the success — and helping the donor families — keeps inspiring you."

Then the woman asked what Jo thought was an odd question: "How do you *feel* about your work?"

Jo began to tell her, and as she did she was surprised that the words that came out of her mouth were so emotional. They were words like "sadness" and "pain." She'd never allowed herself to experience these feelings.

"You feel terrible for these people," she said. "You feel sad yourself, but that's not important because you're serving."

Then something amazing happened. Although she'd been involved in organ procurement for more than three years, Jo had never cried about her work — not in front of a donor family, not even in the quiet of her home. Now as she talked, her eyes misted over and tears began to form. She brushed them away. "Where'd these come from?" she said, forcing a smile.

She looked around the room. All eyes seemed to be on her. She spoke again. "I've never told this before . . . how much this hurt me. I always thought no one except people in my business would understand." Her life, and work, had been built on ambition, efficiency, and achievement, not emotion. She was surprised so much was there.

"You want to help these people . . . to ease their pain. . . ." She almost let go, but held on and composed herself. She left the brunch later that morning and immediately went to see two close friends, Kay and Fern. She could let go in front of them, now that she was beginning to understand what she'd kept inside. She began to tell them about the brunch, and as she did, the lid came off completely. The tears came so hard she shook.

134

Could she do her job if it hurt this much, if she cried this much? She wondered. Didn't this mean she was some kind of sniveling idiot who'd cry all the time, unable to help those who most needed it? Wouldn't crying betray some feminine weakness?

That night at home, Jo wrote a long entry in her personal journal:

> Right at this moment I want to record an unburdening of considerable magnitude. At last to make the connection of the enormous pain I feel daily in my work; the deepest hurt I've carried. It's continually been a part of me, but never mentioned or acknowledged, always growing deeper the more I worked. I'm not afraid of the pain, of going after what matters to these families in the long run. Just that enormous pain I feel because people hurt and I can do so little about it. Nancy pointing out so clearly that I don't communicate this pain to others to have support to lighten it or even acknowledge it.

Suddenly, Jo put down her pen and went to the telephone to call her parents in Tennessee. She was very warm and emotional, and told them of connections she'd discovered in her life. And then she said, "I love you very much," and told them they had meant so much in her life, but she'd never ever gotten around to telling them just how much. Jo then went back to her journal and wrote a final entry.

> Never fearing the pain or wanting to change it because it is *serving people*. They laughed when I said it's really no big deal how much I hurt because I'm serving. I take that as part of the package to serve — you do whatever it takes to serve. I'm just beginning to understand how hard it is to serve . . . but satisfying.

The next several days were both a catharsis and a revelation for Jo. The tears she shed seemed to make up for all the years she'd denied they were there. It awakened her to the pain her work inflicted on her, and how personally she felt the losses of the families. She cried while sitting in her office, reading a letter, having lunch, anytime. More than anything right now, she didn't want to face a donor situation. She was afraid she might collapse. But the pager ran her life, and a call came for her on Wednesday afternoon.

She took the elevator to the Shocktrauma admitting area and walked down the hall. She felt terribly alone as she neared what she knew would be a confrontation with a donor family. She rounded a corner and saw a young wife, curled up on a bench in the corridor. Her husband had just been killed in a car accident. She looked like a child to Jo. Her face appeared stunned. Jo sat down next to her.

"I'm so sorry for what's happened," Jo said.

The young woman nodded, as if to say thank you, but she couldn't speak.

Jo said she knew this was a very hard time, but said, "I'm here to ask you if you'd like to consider donating your husband's organs." As she spoke, Jo began to cry openly.

The woman looked into Jo's eyes. Jo reached to touch her, but the more she tried to comfort her, the more she cried with her.

The woman spoke. She said she wanted to donate her husband's organs. "He was such a good person," she said.

Jo thanked her and told her someday it might help knowing that part of him was living on in someone else.

"I appreciate your talking with me," the young woman said. "It's helped me."

Jo stayed with her for several more minutes, until members of her family arrived.

"Call me anytime," Jo told her.

Jo walked away. She'd discovered something about herself she'd refused to believe for four years: that she could cry and do her job at the same time. No longer did she have to hold back feelings she'd buried deep inside and pretend they didn't exist. Over the next few days, Jo also noticed that the blotches on her hands and arms — what she'd thought was an allergy to the perfusion fluid — seemed to be fading.

It started with a cold on Good Friday, six weeks after Matthew's kidney transplant and three days after he had been discharged from Children's Hospital after his seizure and chicken pox episode. Matthew had always been plagued with allergies and asthma, and when he began wheezing that afternoon, Betty and Jim were not worried. They'd brought him to the clinic at Children's the day before and his kidney-function numbers were fine.

Later that day Matthew developed a slight fever and his breathing rate quickened. They watched him through the evening, put a humidifier in his room, and went to bed at 2 A.M. Jim set the alarm for 3 A.M.

"I'll check him in an hour and you can do the next one," he told Betty.

At three, Matthew's breathing sounded quicker and his forehead felt warm to the touch.

"Sorry, Matthew," Jim said as he woke him up, "I've got to take your temperature."

It was nearly 100 degrees. Jim was relieved it wasn't higher.

He tucked Matthew in, went back to his bedroom, and reset the alarm.

At four, Betty put her hand to Matthew's forehead. He was burning up. His breathing was rapid and shallow. The thermometer read 104 degrees. She ran to Jim, who rushed to Matthew.

Jim took one look at Matthew. "We better get him to Children's."

Betty alerted the hospital. It was too late to awaken family or friends to care for Janie and Valerie, so they wrapped them in blankets and carried them to the car. The girls had witnessed a continuing series of medical crises with their little brother and needed little explanation.

Betty held Matthew tightly in her arms as Jim raced along narrow macadam roads. The girls were now wide awake. Matthew breathed quickly, laboring for air. Jim took quick, nervous glances at him as he drove.

"How's he doing?" he asked Betty.

She put her palm against Matthew's forehead. "He's burning up."

The weeks since Matthew's transplant had been a series of emergencies that blurred with time. Every quiescent period was followed by another emergency. Jim and Betty were never certain whether Matthew was getting better or getting worse. But they endured, their instincts overcoming exhaustion, their fears succumbing to necessity.

Jim glided carefully through red lights and gunned it in the open road. It was a thirty-minute drive from their home to Children's Hospital. This night it took seventeen minutes.

They carried Matthew into the hospital emergency room. Betty stayed to make certain all that could be done was done, then left to take Valerie and Janie home. Jim would stay the night.

X rays showed fluid filling both of Matthew's lungs. Jim looked over the X rays on the emergency room lightbox with one of the doctors. He had learned how to read them.

He looked for the small, fist-sized heart. He couldn't find it, and became convinced the X ray was poor.

"Where's his heart in this?" he asked the doctor.

The doctor pointed to a huge gray area in the middle of Matthew's chest. "This is it here."

"My God, all that?" Jim asked.

Jim couldn't believe it. Matthew's heart looked to be more than double its normal size. The fluid overload that was filling his lungs was also causing a dangerous heart enlargement.

But what was causing the fluid to build up? No one knew, and because they didn't, they couldn't treat it.

The sun rose as the doctors continued to study Matthew. Jim, who had stayed awake all night to comfort his son, listened through the stethoscope and heard the raspy, crackling sounds of diminished lung capacity. Matthew's temperature stayed high; so did his blood pressure.

Later that morning as Jim and Betty sat in a small, brightly lit conference room, a group of physicians seated in chairs around the table talked with them frankly about Matthew. It was a scene to which Jim and Betty had grown accustomed. Paul McEnery was there; so was Dr. Noseworthy, who had transplanted Lisa's kidney into Matthew.

Jim studied their faces. Even Paul McEnery, usually the most optimistic, wore a tight look. In McEnery's kidney-transplant rating system, the fours were the toughest ones. The fives were the ones who didn't make it no matter how hard you tried. The threes were average. They suffered some setbacks, but victory was usually in sight. If there ever were ones and twos in kidney transplants, McEnery had never seen them. Nobody seemed to escape that easily. Matthew was definitely a four, and right now maybe a four plus. Fours kept you guessing and strained your knowledge and intuition to the limit. You were always jockeying with fours, always getting confusing signals from them. Often you weren't sure if they were getting better or worse.

McEnery and the other doctors had looked over all of Matthew's data and had come to a difficult decision. When they explained it, Jim and Betty realized why they looked the way they did.

They wanted to operate because they needed tissue from Matthew's lung to find out what kind of infection he had so they could use the correct drug to treat it.

Jim was appalled. Matthew was too weak to lift his head. How could they operate on him when he was that ill?

McEnery insisted. "If there were any other way to treat Matthew, we'd do it. But there isn't." He explained that sometimes in lung infections the disease organism can be cultured out from coughed-up sputum. But sputum is mobilized by the white blood cells, and Matthew's were suppressed by the antirejection drugs. He had no sputum. Blood cultures would not turn up anything. Surgical biopsy was the only way to get a piece of lung tissue and find out precisely what the infection was. It was another example, when none was needed, of why transplantation was risky; every sneeze, every cut could be a potential threat.

Jim spoke. "You've gotten Matthew this far, so do what you have to do."

Dr. Noseworthy moved next to Betty and put his big, strong arm around her shoulder and gave her a warm hug. Betty was touched by his gesture the same time she was frightened by it. The situation must be just as bad as she imagined.

"I'm going to do the very best I can," Noseworthy told them. "I'm going to control things in there and he's going to come through this."

Given the uncertainties of the situation, that was an extraordinary statement, but it buoyed everyone's spirits.

Betty's eyes misted and Jim felt a surge of optimism.

Jim and Betty returned immediately to Matthew's room to tell him he'd soon go to surgery.

"The doctors have to find out why you have a fever," Betty told him, "so they can give you medicine to make you better."

Matthew studied Betty's eyes. She tried to hide her anxiety.

140

"You're going to be fine, Matthew," she said. "It won't take very long."

The orderlies came to wheel Matthew to the operating room. His temperature was still soaring, his breathing still labored. Jim and Betty held his hands as they moved hurriedly down the corridor, another scene they'd played many times. Jim leaned over the stretcher's safety bars and kissed his son. "You're my little man," he said. "I'm going to see you real soon."

The double doors to the OR suite swung open and Matthew's stretcher disappeared inside. At about the same time, his name was placed on the hospital's critical list.

It was difficult for Jim and Betty to compare the crises that had filled Matthew's short lifetime. Each left its own imprint. But as Jim waited while Matthew was operated on, under the most extreme circumstances, his hope began to ebb. He thought their luck had finally run out. Betty, who'd been careful to guard against optimism anyway, shared his despair.

"We'd better call the folks and let them know what's happening," Jim said.

Betty reached her father. She told him Matthew had just been taken into surgery, and she and Jim would remain at Children's the rest of the day and possibly into the evening, and she made arrangements for her parents to take care of Valerie and Janie.

Betty's parents still lived next door to Jim's parents, and she often took the children to visit them. Her father, who had been partially crippled with polio since his youth, doted on them. So did her mother. Her father had also been a source of inspiration for Betty over the years. No matter the bleakness of the situation, he always found the bright side. He knew Betty was down.

"I know it's hard for you sometimes, honey, but that little boy of yours is going to come out of this, you wait and see. He's going to be good and healthy one of these days."

Betty knew his optimism was real, but she found it hard to share right now. "I hope you're right, Daddy," she said.

Jim spoke briefly with his mother. She told him she was on her way to the hospital to be with them.

Jim's mother, Edna Landis, appeared younger than her early sixties. She and Jim's father had had eight children, but her seventh child, a daughter, was born with a congenitally deformed bowel and lived for only two months. Edna could empathize with Jim and Betty. It was Edna who comforted Betty when she was so devastated after learning she could not donate her kidney to Matthew. She was always there when needed. Jim and Betty called her their "rock."

In the hospital waiting room that was almost a second home to Jim and Betty, Edna read small items from newspapers and magazines to divert their attention. She realized it didn't work. "Let's go into the chapel," she said.

All three walked to the chapel, knelt, joined hands, and prayed for Matthew's survival. Later they went to the hospital cafeteria and tried to eat, but Betty couldn't.

Inside the operating room it was quiet and tense. Noseworthy cut open the middle of Matthew's chest. He had a clear view of his enlarged heart and the pleural cavity around the lungs. He took out a small piece of lung tissue and told the circulating nurse to rush it to the lab. Then he aimed a suction device into the chest cavity and drew out fluid. In someone Matthew's size, two hundred cubic centimeters of fluid in a lung was a lot. Noseworthy found nearly double that. Matthew had nearly died from drowning.

He moved in again with the suction device, pulling out fluid from Matthew's lungs, always careful not to injure the delicate tissues. The more fluid he took out, the more easily Matthew appeared to breathe.

Nearly three hours after surgery began, Jim and Betty heard

Dr. Noseworthy's heavy footsteps. As he entered the room, his face told them the news before words could.

"He's doing just fine," he said. "He came through better than we all expected."

Noseworthy said Matthew had not only tolerated surgery remarkably well, but his temperature was now down under 100 degrees, his heart enlargement was reduced, his lungs were clear of fluid, and his blood pressure was nearly normal.

Jim and Betty embraced. Betty could not stop crying; neither could Edna. All three held on to one another. For Jim, this was the single most joyous moment in all the trials he'd been through with Matthew.

Masked and gowned, all three went to the recovery room. Matthew was in a special, isolated section, hooked up to the intravenous lines and digital monitors that gave instant readouts of his vital signs. All were stable. Dr. Noseworthy had told them a resident doctor was assigned to Matthew throughout the night, and two nurses would stay with him.

Jim kneeled down next to him. "Hey there, my little man. You're doing fine."

Matthew could not speak. His eyes were tired, but they were not beaten, even though he'd just had his seventh major operation in little more than three years. Betty reached over and put Curious George next to him and squeezed his hand to let him feel her presence. "We love you, Matthew," she said, over and over, as he drifted off to sleep.

That evening, in the pathology laboratory, a special silver stain was applied to the small slice of Matthew's lung tissue. Placed under a microscope, the pathologist observed telltale cysts. This was an unequivocal sign that Matthew had pneumocystis, a form of bacterial pneumonia that often attacks immune-deficient people. Matthew was put on the antibiotic Septra.

Day by day, Matthew gained strength. Soon he began painting and laughing at cartoons on television again. His name was taken off the critical list. When he appeared to be completely out of danger, one of the young doctors who'd attended Matthew met Jim in the hall.

"You know, I really didn't think he'd come out of surgery alive," he said.

"Neither did I," Jim answered.

NINE

Shirley Wright's life had not been easy. She hadn't seen her ex-husband — the father of her three children — for nearly three years. During that time, his support for their children, financial and otherwise, had been minimal. Although money was always tight, she did not want to work outside her home when her children were so young. She also realized that much of her paycheck would go for child care expenses anyway. So for now, she lived on money she earned for daytime baby-sitting and on a small amount of state aid. Once the children were older, she planned to go back to work. She had secretarial and accounting skills.

She lived in a small duplex on a narrow residential street. She liked the neighborhood, and so did her children. It was close to a good school and had plenty of young children for them to play with. Her daughter, Elizabeth, had been identified as academically gifted. Now in the sixth grade, she attended advanced classes, had the vocabulary of an eighteen-year-old, and read voraciously. She had already read many of Shakespeare's plays and was now reading a series of books by J. R. R. Tolkien. At first, Elizabeth had regarded Derrick suspiciously because she remembered him as a man who drank too much. But she had grown fond of him. Recently she'd been asking her mother, "Are you going to marry Derrick?"

Shirley always answered noncommittally, and realized that Elizabeth's question was meant as a suggestion.

For a long time, Shirley worried because her sons, Jamaal, four, and Charles, seven, didn't have a man's influence in their lives. After she and Derrick became friends, she was pleased and grateful that he took an interest in the boys, even though he was very limited in what he could do with them.

She realized she was drawn to Derrick at first because she'd seen in him the same unhappiness she'd seen in her own life a few years earlier. He'd been hurt a lot, and so had she. When she was at her low point, alone, broke, with three small children to raise, religion entered her life. It gave her purpose and a new enthusiasm for living.

She realized Derrick's religious commitment was as deep as her own; sometimes she wondered if it was deeper. He'd totally renounced his past life. Friends he once drank with could not even tempt him into having a sip of beer.

Since she'd met him, Shirley had known Derrick did not consider himself attractive to women, or anyone else. "People don't want to look at me," he'd told her. "They see my eyes and turn away." She'd said to him, "People aren't looking inside you. I have, and I think you're beautiful." She had thought he had been hurt too much and too long to believe her. Even now, the eye that had not had the cornea transplant appeared odd. This did not bother Shirley. She had grown comfortable with Derrick and loved him. Within the past two weeks, their long friendship had blossomed into a love affair. Now that she'd crossed that bridge, she had no regrets, and neither did Derrick.

Shirley's phone rang and she went to the kitchen to answer. It was Derrick calling from downtown. Shirley said she'd come pick him up.

It was now early May, and for the past several weeks, Derrick's sight had grown clearer by the day. It was by far the best cornea transplant he'd ever had. His life of diminished expectations seemed to be changing to one of wonderful possibilities. Because he saw so well, he had regained the confidence to seek a job. Although he could live on his $400 a month social security disability check, he now wanted to earn more money, enough so he could contribute something to Shirley and her children. He'd had jobs before. He'd worked in a warehouse for Goodwill Industries and was a school janitor for a while. Both times his sight failed and he couldn't do the job any longer. He believed this cornea would not fail, and he hoped to find a job with a government agency of some kind.

Shirley picked up Derrick and still had time before Elizabeth and Charles came home from school. She always wanted to be there when they arrived.

Derrick went to the living room and read a newspaper. Shortly before Derrick's cornea transplant, an evangelist from Connecticut had visited their church. She told Derrick, "You have a special love for children, and that love will be used by children."

That special love had never been evident before his transplant. When Shirley's children would ask Derrick to play a game with them, he'd always refused. The children didn't understand that he refused because he couldn't see well enough to participate. But since the transplant, the evangelist's "prophecy" seemed to be coming true.

Now Derrick appeared to revel in playing with the children, everything from Monopoly to backyard basketball. On Saturday, he'd promised to take the boys to the Basketball Hall of Fame, just a short distance away in downtown Springfield. Everyone seemed to be excited about it, especially Derrick.

Was the prophecy a "miracle"? All Shirley knew was that her life, and the lives of her children, had been enriched by Derrick, and enriched even more since his sight was restored.

A little after nine, all three children were in bed, and Derrick and Shirley were in her living room. He'd spent a couple of nights with her during the past week, and she invited him again tonight. He wanted to stay.

During the past days, they'd shared their deepest feelings for one another. Shirley told Derrick of the joy she found with him, and Derrick spoke of the gratitude he felt for her. "You saved me," he told her.

As they had many times before, Shirley and Derrick knelt in her living room and prayed for the young girl who donated her cornea, and for her family. Then Shirley reached over and took her Bible off the end table. She opened it to a bookmark at chapter nine in the Gospel According to John. She had read from here often recently, as had Derrick. It was a passage about a blind man whom Jesus came upon.

"Why is he blind? Jesus' disciples asked. Was it caused by the sin of his parents or himself? Jesus answered that it was neither his sin nor his parents' that caused him to be blind, but that the works of God should be made manifest in him. And then Jesus made some mud and placed it over the blind man's eyes and told him to wash in the pool of the Siloam and he went and washed, and came away seeing."

Carolyn Blanchard turned on the small light next to her bed. It was 2 A.M. on a Wednesday in mid-May, more than two months post-transplant. She got up and walked toward a window and looked outside into the darkness, and stood there for a few minutes. It's the hope of every transplant patient that somehow they will be that long shot who escapes unscathed by rejection or any other problem. After nearly two trouble-free months, Carolyn had almost let herself believe she'd be the lucky one. Then she'd noticed the weight gain. It was gradual one day, sudden the next. Then she knew she hadn't escaped.

She walked to the bottom of her hospital bed and picked up her chart, a running chronicle of her medical status, her date of admission, the drugs she took, all her test results, and her daily kidney-function test numbers. Carolyn knew how to interpret her chart. In the dim light, she read it, put it down, and climbed back into bed. Outside her room, she heard the soft footsteps of the nurses walking past. She got up again, picked up her chart, and reread it, as if trying to force the numbers down with her will. She could not sleep. She'd been back at Walter Reed for ten days.

She thought of Tom and the children. How are they doing without me? Will I fight off this rejection, or will I lose this kidney and be on dialysis again? She also worried about their move back to their old home in California. They'd planned it for August, now only three months away. They already had a buyer for their Washington home, but there were scores of details to be worked out. She tried to summon the optimism to ward off her worries, but they kept coming anyway. The night stripped away her defenses.

The hospital stay had been difficult. Several days earlier, Dr. Light had put Carolyn on an experimental immune-suppression drug called Antilymphocyte Globulin, or ALG. Carolyn had taken ALG at the time of her transplant and suffered no serious side effects. However, this time she was struck with a deep, compressing pain in the middle of her chest. It also radiated down her arms. Rushed to the Coronary Care Unit, she was monitored throughout the night. The next day, it was determined she had not had a heart attack, but Dr. Light speculated that because ALG destroys lymphocytes — in the hope that this would stem rejection — it released certain bioactive amines that may have caused a spasm in her coronary artery.

A week after this episode, Dr. Light ordered the same dosage of ALG he'd given Carolyn before. This time, a tape of Nytropaste — a topical form of nitroglycerine absorbed through the skin — was put on Carolyn's chest. It permitted a slow absorption of this drug, which helped open her vessels and prevented spasm. Carolyn was very apprehensive about taking ALG again, but the procedure went well. She had no recurrence of chest pain, but her kidney-function numbers still were slow to respond.

The early morning light brought a respite from worry. Carolyn could hear the hospital's pace quicken. She called home. Tom, an early riser, answered. He asked her how she was doing.

"Not much change," she said. "They're still waiting and watching."

"We knew this rejection was coming," Tom said soothingly. "They told us it was just a matter of time. When they take care of this, things will smooth out."

"I'm still very optimistic," she said. "How are the kids?"

"Greg's up. I'll get him for you."

"Hi, Mom, when are you coming home?" It was a question he asked every time they spoke.

"I'm not sure, honey. They're taking it day by day right now."

During the last couple of days, Carolyn had begun to detect a wistfulness in Greg's voice. There was almost a hint of sadness in it. It always happened when she was away from home.

"How's school going?" she asked.

"Okay, I guess. The best part is there's only a month left till summer vacation."

Carolyn asked about Linda. "She's still sleeping, as usual," he said. Carolyn laughed.

"You take care of yourself, honey. I'll be out of here pretty soon and putting you to work digging up the garden."

Tom came back on the phone. "I'll be over there tomorrow to see you."

She asked him to bring her one of her books on stitchery. He said he would. She passed time in the hospital reading and stitching intricate designs. She was even considering one day starting a stitchery business.

"Love you," Tom said.

"Love you, too," Carolyn answered, hanging up.

A few minutes later, Dr. Light came into her room with a group of other physicians.

"How's everything today?" he asked.

"Pretty well," Carolyn said.

He looked over her chart and palpated her kidney.

"It feels pretty good," he said. "I don't want you to get discouraged. I think you're going in the right direction."

"I won't get discouraged," she assured him.

"I'll see you later," he said, leading the small entourage out of her room.

The days passed and Carolyn's kidney numbers finally came down. As she watched them improve on her chart, she felt her strength and energy return.

During her stay in the hospital for this rejection episode, she had not cried, even during her bleakest moments. She feared if she started, she might not be able to stop. On a Wednesday morning, just a couple of days before her discharge, an orderly brought in her breakfast tray. It had an egg and pieces of shredded wheat, but no bran muffin. Her disappointment was keen.

She asked the orderly to check the breakfast order. He did, but said no bran muffin was mentioned.

"But I always get a bran muffin," Carolyn said.

He left before she could say anything further, and now she began to cry.

Ellen Kelly sat uneasily in the corner of the lawyer's office, shifting her feet and saying nothing. She watched as legal papers were passed back and forth between her parents, the state social worker, and the lawyer. In a few moments, Ellen would be the legally adopted daughter of Eugene and Louise Kelly.

The signing, delayed for nearly two months because of Lisa's death, appeared to bore her. She'd always felt she was a member of the Kelly family. Eugene and Louise had always been Mom and Dad. She felt no tie to her biological parents. Until Lisa's funeral, Ellen's last contact with them had been more than five years earlier. They lived in an old shack deep in the woods, about an hour's drive from the Kelly home. For all her connection to them, they could have lived in China.

Ten years earlier, the social worker had ended Lisa and Ellen's visits to their natural parents because Lisa had become so terrified of the visits, she had to be forced, kicking and screaming, into their home. The Kellys would literally have to pry Lisa's fingers from their car door. It was then that the Kellys undertook formal adoption proceedings.

"Just sign right here," the lawyer said, pointing to the appropriate line.

Louise picked up a pen and inscribed her name, and Eugene did the same.

Louise turned to Ellen and said with a soft smile, "It's official."

Ellen smiled back, but showed little emotion.

Eugene extended his hand to the social worker, a woman in her late forties, and said, "Thank you for all your help."

"Thank you. I wish it could have been a happier occasion," she said.

She turned to Ellen and said, "I'm very happy for you, Ellen . . ." and then her voice trailed off.

They all filed out of the law office. The drive back to the Kelly home was quiet. Louise marked the occasion by making a special roast beef dinner. But what should have been a joyous time instead was quiet and subdued.

Several days later, Ellen did something that made the Kellys concerned. She began wearing Lisa's clothes.

She'd never worn them when Lisa was alive, but now she wore them all the time — to school and with friends on weekend nights. She even had her picture taken wearing one of Lisa's blouses. The fact that she was bigger than Lisa, and the clothes did not fit well, didn't matter to her. Louise considered confronting Ellen, but decided against it. She talked to Maureen about it frequently.

"What do you think it means?" Louise asked.

"I'm as much in the dark as you are, Mom. Maybe it's her way of working something out about Lisa," Maureen answered.

"I keep wondering if I should try and do something about it, try and reach her," Louise said.

"It'll probably pass," Maureen cautioned. "It might be best right now to ignore it and say nothing. I think she'll come out of it."

"I hope you're right," Louise said.

A few days later, Louise and Maureen were at a shopping mall where they met a woman acquaintance. She told Louise and Maureen that she would never permit anyone in her family to donate their organs, and implied Louise shouldn't have either. Louise and Maureen were taken aback, both by the statement and by the woman's insensitivity for making it. It prompted Maureen to write a letter to the local paper. In it, she told how painful the loss of Lisa was for her and her family, but they had gained some measure of solace knowing that her organs were benefiting other people. She concluded, "As my mother once said, 'I only hope that whoever received her eyes, sees the world in the same wonderful way she did.' What more is there to say?"

Indistinct images floated through Jim's mind. A telephone rang . . . a voice spoke. An accident . . . bad accident . . . your daughter's at the hospital . . .

Jim Landis woke up startled. Through the window, he saw a glimmer of spring dawn. It was late May, two and a half months after Matthew's transplant. Jim glanced beside him where Betty slept soundly. A cold, clammy sweat bathed his face and chest. He took a deep breath and thought about his dream. He knew the moment he woke up who it was about. He'd been so consumed with Matthew, lately he'd hardly thought of the family that gave Matthew his kidney. Haunted by his dream, he put his arm around Betty and pulled her close, and tried to find more sleep.

Later that morning, a Saturday, Jim headed to Children's Hospital to see Matthew, as he did every day. Matthew was still there more than two weeks after the surgery that removed the fluid from his chest and determined the source of his lung infection. Jim and Betty each spent about fifty hours a week at the hospital, and Jim worked an additional fifty hours a week at his job. That didn't leave much time for sleep, or anything else.

The obvious signs of fatigue were most evident at work. The repair jobs that usually took him one hour now often took him three. He'd also suffered a rash of injuries. A few days earlier, he'd gashed his leg on a piece of heavy equipment and needed fifty-six stitches to close it. And whenever he was paged for a telephone call, he always felt a tight squeeze in his gut, wondering if this was the call he'd been dreading for three years.

Betty felt the same stresses. She needed Valium to untie the knots in her stomach, and she'd gone back to smoking cigarettes, a habit she'd quit before her first pregnancy.

The stresses Jim and Betty felt were also felt by their daughters. Even the attention showered on them by their grandparents didn't shield them. Nine-year-old Valerie was a fragile, slender brunette with a sensitive face. She was very loving to Matthew, and recently she'd complained of stomach pains at school. A physical checkup revealed no organic problem, but the pains persisted.

Their six-year-old Janie was, on the surface, a smiling, outgoing child, but she had recently begun to wet the bed. She hadn't done that in more than three years.

Jim walked past the nurses' station at Three South. A cluster of doctors, including Paul McEnery, stood there. They were about to begin rounds. Jim checked Matthew's room but couldn't find him. Then he heard a long, loud yell from the hallway.

"Outta the way . . . outta the way," Matthew hollered as he careened down the hall riding in a bright red wagon pulled by another little boy.

"We're the fire truck . . . outta the way," he yelled.

His cheeks were rosy, his eyes alive, his voice strong. He looked up at his father, laughing.

"I see you're feeling pretty well today, Bubby."

"I'm a fireman," Matthew said.

"I can see that," Jim said.

The doctors moved toward Matthew's room. "I think they want to check you over, Matthew. How about getting back in your room?" Jim said.

Matthew hopped out of the wagon and, giggling, ran into his room and hid behind the door.

McEnery played along and pretended not to see him.

"Matthew, where are you?" McEnery asked.

Matthew couldn't restrain himself. McEnery looked behind the door, where all the laughter was coming from.

"There you are," he said, and held Matthew's hand and led him back to his bed.

"I told you this little guy was full of fun, but I'm not sure any of you really believed me," Jim said. "I think you're getting to see the real Matthew now."

"Is that true, Matthew?" McEnery asked. "Are you a funny guy when you're not around all of us?"

Matthew smiled and leaned back on the pillows as McEnery and the other doctors examined him. He grew quieter and held Curious George next to him.

Monica stroked Matthew's forehead.

"Do you want to go home soon?" she asked.

"Yeah," he answered.

"Well, I think you're going to get your wish."

Matthew's eyes lit up. His kidney-function numbers were excellent, and there was no sign of his lung infection. Now more than two months since his transplant, his condition was still day by day, but each day was a little better than the one before it.

At midafternoon Jim, who'd been at the hospital for nearly seven hours, told Matthew he was leaving. Jim worked six-day weeks to keep the family going financially. It cost money even though all of Matthew's medical expenses were paid for by Jim's group health plan at work and Medicare.

"Mommy will be here in a few minutes," he said.

"You go to work?" Matthew asked.

"Yes, Daddy's got to work."

After Matthew's burst of energy in the morning, he'd grown quieter as the day progressed. He was still weak.

"You're going to come home soon, Bubby."

Matthew smiled. " 'Cause I get better."

"Yeah, Bubby, because you've gotten better."

Then Jim leaned over the bed, kissed Matthew, and hugged him. Matthew wrapped his arms around Jim's neck and squeezed as tight as he could.

~~~~~~~~~~~~~~~~~~~ T E N

Jo Leslie downshifted into second gear, popped the clutch, and her VW bus whined and bucked to a stop as the traffic light turned red. Off to her right, a young, helmetless motorcyclist cut into the intersection, slid past a row of slower cars, and roared away.

Jo turned to Fran Danella, sitting in the front seat next to her. "There," she said, "goes a future organ donor."

Fran laughed. So did Bob Grant from the backseat.

It was mid-June and the day was bright and sunny as Jo drove along Green Street on the way to Harbor Place for lunch. They were going to meet Karin Earp there. She was the transplant coordinator at Johns Hopkins Hospital.

For three years prior to her present position, Jo had been an organ-transplant coordinator at Baltimore City Hospitals, and before that she procured organs for the Emory University hospital system in Atlanta. Her present job was her first chance to direct her own program, and she wanted to make it a statewide network that would be a model for the country. That was what she called her "vision," and it was a crucial part of her larger view of her job. But it only added to the pressures she felt.

She also had to keep procuring enough kidneys to satisfy the surgeons at the three Baltimore hospitals who performed kidney transplants and who oversaw her program. She also had to keep her staff happy and functioning, and always she had to deal

157

with donor families. Some type of donor situation occurred nearly every day. Each case meant hours of work. In the first six months of the year, she'd already accrued more than three hundred hours in overtime. Her recent acknowledgment of the pain she'd long held inside had lifted some of her burden. Still, much of the time, she felt emotionally overwhelmed.

"There's one," Fran yelled, spotting a parking place.

"Miracles never cease," Jo laughed as she pulled her bus into the narrow opening.

They walked across the brick terrace toward the American Café. The Baltimore harbor had been transformed from a collection of rundown warehouses and piers into a beautiful array of restaurants and specialty shops that ringed the inner harbor. Across the water the sharp silhouette of the new Baltimore Aquarium stood out against the blue sky. Overhead, seagulls squealed and swooped.

"There she is," Jo said.

They walked quickly up to Karin, a small woman with dark, lively eyes, and Jo hugged her.

They all sat around a table on an outside terrace and ordered sandwiches and a carafe of white wine. As they sat and talked, Jo looked at the sunlight glinting off the rippling water, sipped wine, and began to feel at ease.

"Fran, you've got to tell Karin your story," Jo said.

Fran laughed. "If you insist," she said. A honey-haired North Carolinian, Fran had forged a close friendship with Jo since Fran had been hired two months earlier. They were about the same age, both divorced, and both from the South. "Kindred spirits," Jo said.

Fran took a sip of wine and began her story. She had received a late call to pick up a kidney coming in from Virginia by chartered airplane. It was due to arrive at 5 A.M. at the Baltimore-Washington Airport, and at about four she'd gone to the hospital to pick up the kidney perfusion machine.

The perfusion machine is cumbersome and heavy, about seventy pounds. She had to lug it down six floors to her Datsun. She'd also been up most of the night before on two other kidney placements and was in no mood to be hassled.

"I put the perfusion machine into a wheelchair so I could get it out to my car," she said, "and I'd just opened up the hatchback to put it in when all of a sudden, this hospital security car pulls up and blocks my car. Then this other security guard comes running out of the hospital. He's yelling, 'Wait! wait!' He runs up to me, then in this real sarcastic voice, 'Lady, it's not nice to steal a television set from the hospital.'

"I said, 'What are you talking about?' And then before I have a chance to explain that this isn't a television set, he's threatening to arrest me.

"I was so tired and so mad, I just snapped. I said, 'Look, fella! You take this damn machine and you plug it into any damn socket you can find. And if you get a picture on it, you can even arrest me, okay?'"

"I love it," Karin said, laughing.

"Anyway," Fran continued, "once we'd straightened it out, this security cop just kept apologizing over and over again. I really think I scared the poor guy."

They all laughed again and continued with their lunch, which was interrupted when one of their pagers went off.

"My turn," Jo said.

She left the table, went to a nearby pay phone, and returned shortly. "It was a call from Salisbury," she said. "They've got a twenty-year-old who mashed himself."

"You going?" Fran asked.

"Yeah, and pretty quickly," Jo said. "They've got a surgeon standing by ready to remove the kidneys. They said the family told the doctors they would donate, but they want to talk to me."

Salisbury was three hours by car, which was too far to drive, and there were no scheduled flights available. Jo would have to charter a plane. It was now 2:30, and she realized it would be very late at night before she was back in Baltimore with the kidneys.

The four of them finished lunch quickly and walked to the parking lot. They bade Karin goodbye, and Jo, Fran, and Bob hopped into Jo's VW bus for the short drive back to their office. Within minutes, Jo went from laughing in the warm harbor sunlight to preparing for a flight to a hospital 100 miles away, where she'd confront a distraught family and a young man's death.

Carolyn Blanchard looked in her bathroom mirror and was jolted when she noticed puffiness around her eyes. It was the one symptom that had haunted her for years. She stepped on the bathroom scale and it registered a ten-pound weight gain. When the body starts to reject a kidney, the kidney loses efficiency, more fluid is retained in the tissues, and body weight increases. Carolyn realized this, but as she stood alone and worried in her bathroom, she balanced it against her own tightly held optimism. Maybe it was rejection, but maybe not. Maybe she had too much salt, she thought. That could be it.

It was mid-June, three months since she'd received Lisa Kelly's kidney, and nearly a month since she'd been released from Walter Reed following her first rejection episode. The second one shouldn't happen this fast, she thought. What was going on? She reached down and touched the area of her kidney. It felt a little soft. Was that her imagination? As hard as she tried, her mind couldn't overrule what her body was telling her. She was having another rejection.

Each rejection episode, even when controlled and defeated by drugs, causes permanent damage because the anitbody attack on the transplanted organ leaves scars and diminishes the organ's capacity to perform at a maximum level.

Rejection also causes psychological damage. It creates uncertainty and fear. Rejection was Carolyn's tangible reminder that her link with this new kidney, and the new life it gave her, was a tenuous one. She sat on the cover of the toilet, her face in her hands, praying quietly to herself. She knew what everyone suffering a difficult disease knows, that you fight it alone. Family, friends, doctors, and nurses can help, but in the end you are always alone. She hated being alone.

She heard the bathroom door open slowly and turned to see who was there. She saw Tom's profile through the small opening.

"Get out!" she screamed.

Tom, shocked by the tone of her voice, closed the door quickly and retreated to the bedroom. Carolyn was almost as shocked by her outburst as he was.

When she came out of the bathroom, she told Tom she was sorry.

"I think I've got a problem," she said, by way of explanation. "I'm afraid it's another rejection episode."

Three hours later, Carolyn was waiting on a bench outside Kathy Oddenino's office at the Walter Reed kidney unit. Her blood and urine samples had been taken to the laboratory for analysis. Finally, Kathy Oddenino called Carolyn into her office.

"I guess you know what I'm about to tell you," Kathy said.

"Rejection?" Carolyn asked.

"I'm afraid so," Kathy said. Within an hour, Carolyn was admitted as an in-patient.

Tom came by to see her later that afternoon, but she told him not to come back for a while.

"The kids need you home," she said. "I'll be all right here."

Over the next several days, Carolyn withdrew into herself. Like a wounded animal, she simply wanted to retreat, to be alone. She hardly spoke at all, and when an old friend called,

Carolyn didn't want to see her, didn't even want to talk to her.

"I hope you understand, it's a bad time right now," she explained.

But the optimism that resided so strongly in Carolyn slowly began to emerge. A week later, the world looked more friendly to her, and she called back her friend.

"I'm sorry I cut you off that day. I was feeling down," she explained.

Her friend said she understood and would come by to visit soon.

Carolyn felt better, and her numbers slowly improved. Tom came for regular visits, and she spoke by phone to the children at least twice a day. She began to convince herself that she would lick this rejection.

Dressed in a long pink robe and slippers, Carolyn walked from the hospital library, holding a cookbook and another book on quilting. She was bored by most television shows, so she spent most of her time reading. Outside, it was sunny and hot.

Kathy Oddenino came by to visit, and Carolyn, who felt comfortable with Kathy, shared her feelings. "You get to feel you really aren't carrying your weight when this happens. You know in your head that rejection is all part of it, but I've always been a believer that you can control things with positive thinking. That's why this one's really devastated me. I can't help thinking that I could have prevented it somehow."

"You can't blame yourself for this," Kathy cautioned. "You've got enough to contend with without being so hard on yourself."

"I know," Carolyn said, "I know."

Kathy wished she'd detected more conviction in Carolyn's voice.

Dr. Jimmy Light visited Carolyn every day. He was pleased that this rejection seemed to be waning, but also worried. Her kidney-function numbers were not steady, and he was concerned that the rejection episodes had followed one another so closely.

From the time of the transplant, Carolyn had been especially vulnerable because she'd been on kidney dialysis for five years. The long periods of dialysis had weakened her body, sapping it of the strength she needed to hold her own against prolonged rejections. Light thought it would take a lot of work over the next several months to give Carolyn a good chance of keeping her kidney. He did not want her to move to California, as she was now planning to do in August.

"I'd like to have you around here so we can keep an eye on you," he told Carolyn one afternoon.

She thanked him for his concern and told him she genuinely trusted him and the care she received at Walter Reed. "But I just can't leave my family again," she said. "They need me and I have to be with them."

"Could you stay a few months, then go out there when this has settled down?" he asked.

"I just couldn't," she told him. It wasn't that Carolyn disregarded her health; it was simply that the sense of duty, and love, she felt for her family was so powerful. The idea of a separation brought back memories of leaving them in Korea, and she'd vowed never to do that again, and she was keeping that vow.

Light recognized her mind was made up and pressed her no further.

Two days later Tom visited, announcing, "Happy anniversary," as he walked into her room to hand her a bouquet of roses.

"Happy anniversary to you, too," she said smiling. Tom leaned over and kissed her. They'd been married the day he'd been graduated from West Point, exactly twenty years earlier. They had planned to make a special day of it. Instead, Tom sat on the edge of the bed and shared Carolyn's hospital lunch with her, right off the tray. Their anniversary dinner was tasteless chicken breast and overcooked broccoli.

"You like the cuisine and fancy china?" she kidded.

"Nothing but the best," he laughed.

He opened a small box that held a white cake with the words *Happy Anniversary* on it, and they both had a generous piece.

Tom said Greg and Linda were both doing well, and they were helping him prepare for their move. "We're packing boxes every day," he said, "and getting some of the stuff ready for the garage sale. We sure have collected a lot of things over the years."

"I wish I could be there to help," Carolyn told him.

"Just get over this rejection," he said. "That's all the help we need."

Carolyn studied Tom's face as he sat on the edge of her bed. It appeared drawn, with a trace of sadness.

She'd been worried about him the past few weeks. He was extremely tired all the time. Recently, he'd stood on a ladder to hammer a nail, and after a couple swings, he had become so exhausted he had to step down and rest. He'd been through a battery of tests at Walter Reed, but physiologically he was given a clean bill of health. The doctors suspected his fatigue might be stress-related, a reaction to his forced retirement from the military. There was also some suspicion that it had something to do with Carolyn, and not just his obvious concern with her health.

Carolyn no longer needed Tom to run her home dialysis machine. To some extent, that also meant that she needed Tom less.

Doctors had observed that in some people, this situation caused depression, even a sense of loss — of feeling less needed, and therefore less loved. Sometimes this feeling manifested itself in the form of physical complaints and actual disorders.

The doctors had talked to Tom about it, and he'd told them the same thing he'd told Carolyn. "I've looked into myself as deeply as I can, and I don't have any sense at all that I feel that way. The day I learned I no longer had to run that dialysis machine was one of the freest days of my life, like I just had gotten out of jail. As far as I can tell, there's not even the tiniest part of me that wants to go back to that."

His fatigue persisted.

Over the next few days, Carolyn's kidney function improved, and this second rejection was brought under control. She went home in early July. Her two rejection episodes had caused her to spend Mother's Day, Father's Day, Memorial Day, her anniversary, and the Fourth of July in the hospital.

But July would not be an easy month for Carolyn. They were planning to move back to California in early August, so much of the month was spent packing and attending to the scores of other details involved in moving. She was also visiting the clinic twice a week. Even Carolyn's renewed energy and resolve were being tested.

Matthew's voice was weak and distant. "Mommy," he cried. Betty and Jim began searching their house to find him. They looked in his bedroom, in closets, behind the sofas and chairs, under the beds. Again, his little voice cried out, "Mommy."

"Where in God's name is he?" Jim said. He was beginning to panic. When Jim was a little boy, his sister had fallen into a vent opening and had slid from the second floor of their home all the way down to the cellar. He feared Matthew might be caught in a large pipe or vent of some kind.

"Mommy," Matthew cried out again.

"Where are you, Matthew? Tell us!" Betty shouted.

They raced downstairs together. Matthew cried out once more, and Jim got a fix on it.

"The dryer!" he said.

Betty opened the dryer door and there, curled up in a tight ball, was Matthew. He began to giggle, then laugh, then howl.

"You couldn't find me," he said between laughs.

Perhaps they should have been angry at Matthew, perhaps with a healthy child they would have been. But when they found him, their only emotion was great relief.

"Bubby," Jim asked, "what are you trying to do, scare us to death?"

Matthew gave them a quick look, then ran off. "I guess his sense of humor is back," Jim said.

Matthew had been discharged from Children's Hospital in late May, and since then he had grown steadily stronger. In early July, he had his fourth birthday party in his backyard. He'd celebrated with presents, including coloring books, trucks, new paints, and a chocolate cake that had a big number 4 on the top.

Betty brought him to the clinic at Children's twice a week, where he was always greeted like visiting royalty. His Dutch-boy haircut highlighted his round, cherubic face, and his brown eyes sparkled with a vitality his illness had long suppressed. During the clinic visits, he ran around, hid, peeked around corners, and otherwise stayed in perpetual motion. Everyone there indulged him. They let him sit at their desks and gave him paper and pencils to sketch with.

Monica could still draw blood without causing Matthew to cry, and during his visits she always called down to the lab to tell Betty the results before he left for home. Week after week, the same answer came back: Matthew's kidney-function numbers were holding steady; there were no signs of rejection.

This seemed to happen so gradually that there was no single moment, or day, or week, when it occurred to everyone that Matthew might really be getting better, that he just might be past the critical stage. Monica thought to herself that he'd had a long run of good numbers, which was something he'd never done before. And as the weeks passed into late July, she began to let herself believe this was indeed the beginning of a new beginning.

On a Friday at the end of July, nearly five months after his transplant, Jim and Betty both took Matthew to the clinic. Matthew was given the usual tests, and then Jim and Betty asked to speak with Dr. McEnery. McEnery led them to a quiet corner of the clinic and they sat down.

Jim spoke first. "We haven't been on a vacation since Matthew was born, and we're thinking of driving up to Wisconsin for about ten days in August."

Betty said their major worry, of course, was Matthew. Although he looked and acted well, they feared being too distant from Children's for too long a time. "We don't want to jeopardize anything," she said.

McEnery told them he understood their worries, that any parents who'd been through what they'd been through would feel the same way. But he said Matthew had been doing exceedingly well. His numbers were close to sensational, and there were no symptoms of any other problems. It was his experience, he said, that after the initial turmoil of a kidney transplant begins to quiet down, the chances for long-term success brighten considerably.

And then McEnery looked directly at Jim and Betty and told them something they had never heard before. "I think you'd better begin to realize you have a healthy son. Take your vacation. Enjoy yourself and don't worry about every little thing. I think he'll do just fine."

Jim and Betty thanked McEnery, and Jim admitted he was a bit stunned. "It's just that no one has ever said that to us before," Jim said, "and I guess I never thought the day would come when a doctor would say that."

"Well, I said it," McEnery said, "because it's true."

Betty and Jim had endured nearly four years of almost constant medical crises with Matthew. They'd always known Dr. McEnery to be a straight shooter with them. He'd told them the truth even when they might not have wanted to hear it. Now he'd told them their little boy, who five months earlier was running out of time because he was losing all kidney function, who less than three months earlier was in a seizure from which they feared he might never regain consciousness, who then was exposed to a potentially lethal herpes virus, who was then hit with a bacterial infection that filled his lungs and nearly cost his life again, was healthy.

Jim and Betty immediately began planning a trip to Wisconsin. They wanted to visit some old friends in Sheboygan and then drive up to Door County in the northern part of the state, one of the most picturesque areas in America. Betty also began calling nursery schools. It had seemed unimaginable to her just a few weeks earlier, but she was making plans for Matthew to attend nursery school in the fall.

On a warm day in August, a day when Matthew seemed especially exuberant, Betty took him to a nearby park and watched him play in the grass. He ran and laughed, dug in the dirt, and sat on the swing. The day was perfect; it seemed suspended in time. She sat in the cool shade under a tree and Matthew came over to her and crawled into her lap. She put her arms around him and kissed him. As she held her little boy, who for three years had been in nearly constant peril, she thought how happy he was, how happy she was, and how profoundly grateful she was to the family who made it possible. If she could, she would have picked Matthew up in her arms and brought him to them to show what they had done for him.

Although Ellen Kelly had stopped wearing Lisa's clothes, much to the relief of Eugene and Louise, she still did not talk about her sister. She hadn't even mentioned her since shortly after the accident, and the Kellys remained troubled by her silence. By all outward appearances, she was doing fine. A part-time job at a local supermarket gave her spending money during the summer, and she had a large circle of friends, all of whom Louise liked.

Ellen, now nearly sixteen, returned to high school in September. She'd never been a top student, but she did well enough to get by, and she had never caused any problems in school. That's why Eugene and Louise were so surprised when the school called them to say Ellen had been taken to the principal's office for setting off a firecracker in the school hallway.

Louise was troubled by the incident, but more by the way Ellen had done it. She'd lit the firecracker in full view of a number of people. When Louise spoke to Ellen about it, Ellen only wanted to forget it.

"I didn't think anyone would get all that excited by one firecracker," she said.

That seemed to put an end to it, but a couple of weeks later, Louise received another call from the school. This time Ellen had been caught smoking in the girls' room, and Ellen didn't even smoke. This incident was similar to the first in one important respect: it was done in plain view of many people. The principal told Louise that if there was another incident, he would have to suspend Ellen from school for a couple of days.

"I think I ought to ask the school psychologist to see her," Louise told him.

The principal said that was a good idea. "I'll have my office make the request," he said.

That night Louise told Eugene, "It's so obvious to me that she wants to get caught."

"Sounds like she wants attention," he said.

Ellen grew more subdued and withdrawn after the smoking incident, and one morning Louise kept her home from school. "I want you to take a day off," Louise told her.

In the late morning, as both were in the kitchen preparing

169

lunch, Louise approached the subject of professional help. "I've spoken to the principal about a school psychologist," she said. "I thought you might like to talk to one."

Ellen busied herself with making a sandwich and didn't answer.

"He might be able to help you with what's bothering you," Louise said.

"Nothing's bothering me," Ellen said firmly.

"I just thought —"

"I'm okay," Ellen interrupted. "I don't need to talk to any psychologist."

Ellen's back was turned to Louise, and Louise noticed that Ellen stopped whatever she was doing and stood motionless for several seconds, as if collecting her thoughts. She then turned and looked directly at her mother. "I want to talk to you," she said, "not to some psychologist."

Louise moved directly to her, and Ellen began to sob. "You don't know how much I hurt," she said.

Louise wrapped her arms around her daughter, held her tightly, and spoke quietly to her. "Tell me, honey. I want you to tell me."

Ellen began to speak of her pain and the sadness she carried around inside her since Lisa's death. "I couldn't even talk about it," she said. "I felt so alone. Lisa always understood me. She always knew how I felt."

"I know she did. I know how much you loved her, and how much you miss her," Louise said.

Ellen rested her head on Louise's shoulder. "I could never stay mad at her, not even when we had a fight," Ellen said.

"I could never stay mad at her either, she was just so good. You know, honey, I ache inside, too," Louise told her. "And I cry all the time about her. I just didn't ever want you to see me crying. I thought it would make you sadder. I guess I should have let you see me. It's good to let it out."

As they stood alone in the kitchen, embracing one another, they shared feelings and memories of Lisa they'd never spoken of before.

That morning marked a change in Ellen, gradual at first, but steady. She was able to talk openly of Lisa. She could even laugh at some of the funny moments they'd shared.

That morning also marked a change for Louise, a step toward a deeper reconciliation with Lisa's death, and with Ellen. The distance she had sensed between herself and Ellen had been real, and now that it was out in the open, it had begun to evaporate.

Each member of the Kelly family in his or her own way was trying to cope with Lisa's death.

For Maureen, reconciliation came partly in the form of a dream. In it, Lisa was dressed in a flowing white gown, and her hair had grown out longer. She seemed to walk right up to Maureen's bedside. She appeared so real to Maureen that she felt her presence in her bedroom. Then Lisa spoke, in her soft, sure voice. "I'm all right," she said. "I'm doing fine. . . ." And the dream ended.

ELEVEN

It was 4 A.M. on a Tuesday in October. Carolyn stirred and woke. As she'd done the past several nights when she had awakened, she slipped into her robe and went into the kitchen. She made a cup of herbal tea for herself and sat down at the kitchen table to read, hoping she'd soon be sleepy again.

The move from Washington to California had gone smoothly, but once in California, Carolyn and her family had been nagged by a number of problems. Greg and Linda were enrolled in schools that Carolyn did not believe to be academically sound, and their home, located on a pleasant, tree-lined street in an older Los Angeles suburb, needed work. All through late August and September, Carolyn had felt fatigued. At first she thought it was from the long drive and all the work involved in the move, but even when she rested it grew worse. She'd wake up tired in the morning, by noon she'd be dragging, and in the evening after dinner she'd fall asleep on the living room sofa. The fatigue was as bad as it had ever been on dialysis.

She took fourteen pills a day and went to a medical clinic at a nearby military hospital once a week where blood was routinely drawn. During September, her kidney-function numbers had risen steadily, and it was clear she was rejecting her kidney once again. Her blood pressure had also risen.

Carolyn's California physician was a career military doctor. He was pleasant and friendly to her, and he recognized she was in rejection. He treated her by increasing her steroids, but Carolyn's kidney-function numbers and blood pressure were not lowering, nor was her fatigue lessening.

In late September she had been admitted to the hospital for treatment of a rejection that had most likely been going on for days, if not weeks.

The brief hospital stay had not significantly improved her condition, so in early October she kept waking up at night, knowing she would have to decide soon whether or not to go back to Walter Reed. By mid-October, seven months after her transplant, feeling saturated with steroids and showing no improvement in her kidney-function numbers, she called Dr. Light.

"I want to get back there for an evaluation, as quickly as you can see me," she told him.

"Come as soon as you can," he said.

In less than a week, Carolyn was back at Walter Reed. Dr. Light found Carolyn's kidney-function numbers dangerously high. Her creatinine was three times normal, and her BUN level was eight times normal.

He took a needle biopsy of her kidney tissue, and when the small sliver of tissue was examined under the laboratory microscope, it appeared pale. A closer look showed the kidney's delicate blood-vessel network was badly scarred by the antibody attack. The message was plain: Carolyn was in chronic, irreversible rejection that was slowly destroying her donor kidney. There was no realistic hope of keeping it. It could take weeks or even months, but sooner or later it was definitely going to quit.

"I'm still hoping," she told Dr. Light when he broke the news. "Maybe this kidney can keep me going for a while, maybe a few months, or even a year or two."

Dr. Light thought that was unrealistic, but he tried to appear optimistic. "We'll hope for the best," he said.

By late October, all tests and treatments were completed. Feeling stronger, Carolyn returned to California.

It was ten o'clock on a Friday night in early November, and Jo Leslie couldn't believe what she was hearing over her kitchen telephone. The on-call surgeon, the one assigned to go out and remove kidneys from donors this night, was refusing to go.

Jo, her heart racing and temper rising, did everything she could to control herself.

"I think it's imperative that we go now," she said. "Bob Grant's been in Cumberland since yesterday on this, and he's exhausted. There's no one at that hospital who can remove the kidneys."

The surgeon remained unmoved. "Schedule it for the morning. I've had a hard week."

I've had a hard week, too, but that doesn't mean I don't do my job, Jo thought. She tried another tack. "We're not sure how stable the patient is . . . they could lose her before morning."

The surgeon's voice was flat and unemotional. "I'll go in the morning, and that's that."

He would not budge and Jo gave up trying. "Would it be all right with you if I found another surgeon who could go there tonight?" she asked.

"It's fine with me," he answered.

"Goodbye," she said, and slammed the phone down hard.

"Damn!" she shouted to no one as she tried to collect her thoughts. She couldn't believe a doctor, especially one who transplanted kidneys, would leave her in the lurch like this.

The day before, Cumberland Hospital had called. There had been an automobile accident involving a mother, father, and their young daughter. The young girl was killed instantly, the mother suffered irreversible brain damage, and the father, multiple injuries and a concussion. He had survived.

Bob Grant had been in Cumberland for almost forty-eight hours waiting for the husband to regain consciousness so he could ask his permission to remove his wife's organs. A few minutes before Jo had called the doctor, Bob had called her to say that he'd gained permission. He was now so emotionally and physically exhausted that he had also asked her to come with the surgeon to relieve him.

Jo paced up and down and tried to swallow her anger. She had to think clearly, and she knew finding a surgeon would be difficult. There were surgeons at three Baltimore hospitals, University, Johns Hopkins, and Baltimore City, who had experience in removing kidneys for transplant. The surgical departments of these three hospitals oversaw Jo's organ-procurement program and had the ultimate authority for it. Jo knew most of these surgeons well.

She got on the phone and started working her way down the list. For one reason or another, surgeon after surgeon was unavailable. One was out of town, another was ill, another had been up forty hours straight and had just gone to bed. "If you can't find anyone else, I'll go. But I'm so tired I can't keep my eyes open, so I don't know how much help I'd be," he told Jo.

Finally, she paged Dr. Melville Williams, the head of kidney transplantation at Johns Hopkins.

"I'm involved in a case right now and I can't break away," he told her.

"How long will you be tied up? I've tried everyone," Jo said.

"If it clears up soon, I'll call you back," he promised.

He was her last hope. Jo made herself a cup of instant coffee and tried to read while she waited for the phone to ring. Twenty minutes later it did.

"I can go," Williams said.

"I'll meet you in front of Hopkins in a half hour," Jo told him.

She called the charter service at the airport, then raced over

175

to her office, picked up the Styrofoam cooler, and drove over to Hopkins. Williams was standing in front of the hospital entrance, and he hopped into her VW bus.

"I'm not too thrilled with some members of your profession tonight," she said.

"What happened?" he asked.

She told him about the reluctant on-call surgeon as they drove toward the airport.

An hour later, the twin-engine plane made a steady, westward course toward Cumberland. Jo looked out of the window at the stars and moon. It was a cold, clear night, and she'd seldom seen them shine so brightly. The land two thousand feet below was almost totally dark, broken only by the occasional lights of a moving car or an isolated home. It was now midnight. Jo guessed she was somewhere over West Virginia.

The 135-mile flight took about an hour, and Jo spent that time going over the task that lay in front of her, ticking off the procedural steps she'd take when they landed. She felt the plane gradually descend and recalled her first flight to Cumberland the previous spring. It was daytime then and she was entranced by the beauty of the Allegheny Mountains that ringed the city. Now as she looked out into the vast darkness, the thought of those mountains unnerved her.

Jo and Dr. Williams were met at the airport terminal by hospital security guards, who drove them directly to the hospital. They both headed immediately for the operating room, where the donor had already been taken. On a bench outside the OR, Jo saw Bob Grant. A priest was sitting next to him. Bob's exhausted eyes lit up when he saw Jo.

"You did great. I know this one was very tough," Jo told him.

Bob eyed Dr. Williams, who he knew wasn't on call, and Jo said, "I'll tell you about it later."

"Everything's set. The husband signed the donation forms," Bob assured her.

"How's he doing?" Jo asked.

Bob shrugged his shoulders. "He's doing better medically. He's got a lot of family around the area. They were with him all day."

"I gotta go. You get some sleep," Jo shouted over her shoulder as she ran for the OR.

Jo and Dr. Williams changed into surgical greens and scrubbed. Although it was nearly one in the morning, a group of doctors and nurses had waited so they could witness the surgery. Jo stood on a small stand to the side of the operating table and held retractors at the ready. Williams, a fast and skilled surgeon, began the kidney removal. It was nearly dawn before both kidneys were out. Jo packed them in the cooler.

She thanked the doctors and nurses for calling her about the donor. "I really appreciate it. It'll mean a lot to some other people," she said.

Then she and Williams left for the airport, where the charter plane awaited them. Early into the flight, Jo could see the brightening horizon in the distance. She tried to sleep, but the engine noise, her thoughts, and the intensity of the night kept her awake. Even before tonight's incident with the on-call surgeon, she'd felt buffeted by the strains of her work. She'd begun to wonder how much longer she could do it.

Through the summer, and into the fall, she'd noticed changes in herself. She often felt weary and fatigued. Friends began to remark that she seemed withdrawn. They even accused her of losing her sense of humor. And the splotches on her hands and arms had gotten worse again.

At work, she had found it difficult at times to get herself up psychologically to face a donor family. It had always been the most trying part of her job, but also the most satisfying. Now she sometimes found herself facing it with a sense of dread.

In the past, when she'd had misgivings about her work, she'd glossed over them with a quip. But now the jokes didn't hide the fact that after four years of dealing with grief and death on a regular basis, especially the sudden, violent death of young people, it seemed to be catching up with her.

Recently, on a day her job seemed especially difficult, she'd turned to Fran and said, "Sometimes I think I just need to be with people who aren't all dead."

Her workload had become simply overwhelming. By November, she'd accrued more than 500 hours of overtime, and more and more she had begun to feel she had no private life. Everywhere she went it seemed her pager sounded. It interrupted dinner parties, movies, sleep, and once it called her out of the sauna at her athletic club where she tried to exercise away the tensions of her work. Each time it sounded, she knew it might mean hours of work.

The plane banked sharply as it began its approach, and Jo saw the familiar landscape of the Baltimore-Washington Airport off to her left. The cooler was close by her side. Fifteen minutes later, she drove toward Baltimore, and sharp memories of the incident with the on-call surgeon the night before emerged. She grew angry and disillusioned. Her work depended on surgeons, and she had taken care to develop good relationships with most of them. She wondered if this incident might cause that to change, and more important, she wondered if it would cause her to change. Her work needed the right mix of enthusiasm and dedication, both from herself and from the medical professionals she worked with. If any of that were lost, her work would be impossible.

She arrived back at her office, still running on adrenaline. The kidneys had already been tissue typed with blood samples obtained the day of the accident. Now Jo scanned the computer printout of potential recipients. After a long morning of telephone calls, she placed the kidneys with recipients in Tennessee and Texas. Then she went home to bed.

It was late November and Betty was in the bathroom when she heard a steady tapping noise coming from outside the door.

"What are you doing out there, Matthew?" she hollered.

"I'm fixing the door," Matthew answered.

The tapping sound continued for a few moments, then it stopped. Betty pushed the door open as she left the bathroom and felt it leave her hand, then it crashed to the floor. She was stunned as she looked down at the door. She turned to Matthew, who was standing in the hallway. He looked surprised, too, but there was also a look of satisfaction, and he quickly dissolved into laughter. Soon he was laughing uncontrollably, and Betty joined him as she looked down and saw the door-hinge pins next to his hammer.

Matthew's "fixing" was almost nonstop. A few days later, as Jim lay in bed, half asleep, he heard the sound of a hammer. What now? he thought to himself.

"Is that you, Matthew?" he called out.

"Yeah."

"What's all that pounding?"

"I'm fixing the wall."

Jim jumped out of bed. By the time he reached the living room, he found Matthew pounding his third hole in the living room wall. Jim was remodeling the living room and he removed some wall sections, but not where Matthew had just punched three new holes.

"Bubby," Jim said, trying to control himself, "I didn't want any holes there."

Matthew looked at his father, and Jim realized he wasn't going to punish him.

"Daddy needs help over here," he said, showing Matthew the wall he was knocking down. Matthew walked over and began pounding.

Matthew's recovery continued to be remarkable. As he grew more active, Jim and, especially, Betty had to restrain themselves from slowing his activity down. They wanted him to live as normally as he could. But that still hadn't kept Betty from wincing every time she saw Matthew running in the yard or climbing up a tree. Only recently had she begun to relax a bit.

He had developed minor respiratory problems, which at first concerned Betty and Jim. They suspected, however, that it was only an allergy, and after they gave their cat away, Matthew's respiratory problems eased, which seemed to confirm their theory. Since the summer, Matthew had grown nearly three inches and was now approaching normal height for a four-year-old. He seemed to be overcoming a problem in kidney transplantation among young children that had frustrated doctors for years. The steroids needed to combat rejection also suppressed growth. In effect, this defeated one of the major goals of kidney transplantation, which was to give the child a normal, healthy life.

Recently, Dr. McEnery and his colleagues at Cincinnati Children's Hospital had discovered that by giving steroids every other day, instead of every day, children could grow normally and still ward off rejection. Dr. McEnery had announced these findings before a meeting of transplant specialists. "I don't know why it works," he'd said. "All I can tell you is that it does work."

Matthew was one of his best examples. He'd had no further problems with rejection, and his growth was accelerating. The tapering off of the steroids also meant that Matthew's face thinned down to a more normal size.

Jim and Betty were not counting days, but they were aware of the passage of time. It had been more than eight months since Matthew's transplant. He still went to the clinic once a week, but these visits were now becoming routine.

Jim and Betty did continue to worry about the long-term psychological effect Matthew's medical experience would have on him. The doctors had told them that it would probably not be a problem, but sometimes Matthew would pinch Jim or Betty — try to hurt them — and they thought this might be a result of suppressed anger from his hospitalization.

But mostly, they only saw a normal, exuberant four-year-old. He had never complained when he was ill and did not complain now, nor did he talk about his past illness. Betty often wondered what he did remember about it, but did not attempt to discuss it with him.

One day in late November as she cleaned Matthew's room, Betty found a color photograph under Matthew's bed. It had been taken in the hospital earlier that year. In it, Matthew was surrounded by some of the doctors and nurses who had cared for him. They were smiling, and Matthew, as was often .ae case back then, was looking forlorn.

What really puzzled Betty was a tear in the photo or, more accurately, a hole about the size of a dime, which had been punched right out of it and appeared to have been done deliberately. Then Betty realized what was missing from the photo: Curious George. Someone had quite intentionally ripped George out of the picture!

Curious George had been such a fixture in Matthew's room, Betty only noticed then for the first time that he wasn't in his normal place next to Matthew's pillow. She searched Matthew's room and found George in one of his closets, hidden out of sight in a corner.

~~~~~~~~~ TWELVE

Tom parked the car in the hospital parking lot, walked around to open the passenger door, and took Carolyn's hand.

"Are you all right?" he asked.

"I think I've got myself under control," she answered.

It was the end of her kidney, and the redness of her eyelids told much of what she felt. The kidney had limped along during the six weeks since she'd been discharged from Walter Reed, but now it was totally ravaged by antibodies and barely functioning.

All through November, Carolyn had seen the signs of decline in the fluid that filled her tissues and in the weight gain this had caused. She'd also seen it in the rising numbers on her chart every week at the clinic. But the irrevocable sign had come yesterday when the kidney ceased making urine. Now, in this first week of December, she faced the most devastating consequence of its failure. She had come to the hospital to go back on "the machine" that she so hated and now so desperately needed.

It was a warm, sunny California day, too nice for such a bad time, she thought. Although Carolyn refused to feel sorry for herself, she couldn't help but feel this was a defeat for her. Despite that, she searched for the bright side. "No matter what has happened to this kidney," she said as they walked, "it got us through the move from Washington and helped us get the kids settled here. If I'd been on dialysis all that time, these things would have never gone as well as they did." She also realized Tom was feeling stronger now, and the problems that had caused his physical weakness seemed to be ebbing.

Tom and Carolyn walked hand-in-hand into the military hospital and toward the kidney unit. Carolyn remained composed and even smiled at some familiar faces as they walked down the corridor. She slipped into an examining room near the dialysis area, and a young doctor who had treated her during the past several weeks walked in. Carolyn greeted him cheerfully.

"I'm really amazed at you," he said. "I thought you would be falling apart."

It was the wrong thing for Carolyn to hear. Her false cheerfulness dissolved in an instant. "You weren't supposed to say that," she said. She buried her face in her hands and wept.

The doctor walked over to pat her on the back, but Carolyn, this most courteous of women, would have none of it.

"Don't pat me on the back!" she yelled. "Just leave me alone!"

Carolyn kept her promise to Tom: she did not go back on home hemodialysis. Within a few days of her kidney failure, she underwent minor surgery to implant a small plastic access tube into her peritoneal cavity, so she could begin Continuous Ambulatory Peritoneal Dialysis (CAPD). CAPD was a new form of self-administered dialysis that would replace hemodialysis. She could do it herself at home. Rather than cleanse her blood of waste products by filtering, as in hemodialysis, CAPD relied on osmosis. Four times a day, Carolyn poured two liters of special sterile cleansing fluid called dialysate into her peritoneum — the abdominal and pelvic cavity that is sealed by a membrane — through the access tube. It remained there for four hours while it drew the impurities from her blood and tissues, then she drained it out and replaced it with more dialysate.

It was hardly the same as having her own kidney, but she soon realized she had a much higher energy level than she had had on hemodialysis. Also, her food and fluid restrictions were less stringent than they had been on hemodialysis. The only drawback was the potential for infection around the site of the implanted tube, which Carolyn was careful to prevent.

CAPD worked so well that by Christmas, Carolyn felt strong enough to travel by car to Oregon with Tom and the children to visit her mother, who lived alone in a retirement community there. Carolyn's father, a retired fireman, had died five years before. During the drive, they stopped at a restaurant in northern California one evening, where Carolyn performed a dialysis exchange in the backseat of the car. Carolyn had put on a surgical mask and begun draining the fluid, when a couple pulled up in their car and parked right next to them. They got out and peeked over at Carolyn, then said something to each other that Tom overheard.

"What did they say?" Carolyn asked.

"The woman said, 'The only thing I can figure out is that she's having a baby,' " he answered.

By January, a low-grade fever that Carolyn had periodically been running grew more persistent. She also felt nauseated frequently and had developed a cough. When Kathy Oddenino called Carolyn from Walter Reed, she told Carolyn that it sounded to her as if the donor kidney had become infected.

"I think you ought to come back here again, Carolyn, so we can take a look at you," Kathy told her.

In late January, for the second time in three months, Carolyn returned to Walter Reed, where tests confirmed that the transplanted kidney was infected. In early February, eleven months after the kidney transplant, the scarred and shrunken kidney was removed.

At the end of February, still on CAPD, Carolyn was released from Walter Reed. Her hair had been thinned by the steroids, but the puffiness in her face was gone, and she looked and felt better. Before she left, she told Kathy that she did not want her name placed on the transplant computer right now, because she didn't want to put herself and her family through the ordeal again so soon. "So much happened this year," she said. "You look back at a year like this and you wonder how you got through it at all."

A friend came to the hospital to drive Carolyn to Dulles Airport. As they drove, Carolyn told her that even though she had lost the kidney, she still often thought of the young girl who'd given it to her and of her family. "Losing the kidney doesn't diminish what they did for me, or how grateful I'll always be. I feel terrible that they had to suffer this loss so I could have a kidney. But I'm glad I tried the transplant. You've always got to try."

The Dulles Airport passenger terminal loomed in the distance, and Carolyn's mind turned to dialysis. "I dialyzed myself on the flight out here. I just went into the restroom and did it," she said. Then she laughed. "I suppose all those other passengers must have wondered what I was doing in there so long."

The car pulled up directly in front of the terminal, and Carolyn smiled and said in a strong voice, "I'll keep on fighting. There's a lot of life left in me yet. Remember, I've got to raise those kids."

She waved goodbye and moved into the line of passengers, her dialysis equipment at her side, waiting to board her flight back home.

185

It was Sunday morning and Matthew, dressed for church, preened in front of his bedroom mirror. He wore a sport coat, blue shirt, red tie, polished shoes, and brown pants with a sharp crease.

Betty and the girls said they needed a couple more minutes. "But I'm ready," Matthew announced.

"You sure are, Bubby," Jim said. "You're all slicked up."

That he was. He looked so healthy, there was not even a hint that he had ever been ill a day in his life. He was growing so fast that Betty had trouble keeping him in clothes.

As they drove to the Faith Lutheran Church, the same church they'd attended for years, Matthew sat in the backseat between his two sisters. They had stopped mothering him as they had when he was ill. Now they treated him like a little brother, meaning he was sometimes adorable to them, but mostly a pest.

For Jim and Betty, caring medically for Matthew now meant making certain he took his pills each day and getting him to the Children's Hospital clinic once a week. At every clinic visit the results were the same: kidney-function numbers were normal; blood pressure, normal; white count, normal; red count, normal; hematocrit level, normal. They never tired of hearing it.

The Landises arrived a few moments before the service began. The five of them slipped into a pew near the back. The girls sat quietly with Matthew between them.

In the front of the church was an array of beautiful flowers. Jim and Betty picked up a mimeographed copy of the day's church program and looked through it. Jim's eyes were riveted to the bottom of the page, where it said: *"Flowers in Memory of Matthew Landis's donor."*

Jim recognized the work of his mother. Then it struck him: it was a year to the day since Lisa Kelly's death, and a new life for Matthew. They had made it to this magic milestone. As Jim

186

looked at the dedication, and then at the yellow, pink, and white flowers, all the joys, sorrows, and gratitude he'd felt for Matthew, for Lisa, and for Lisa's family welled up inside him. He turned to look at Betty. She was crying, too.

Sunday supper was finished, the dishes washed and put away, and Maureen couldn't keep her eyes off her kitchen clock. Lisa's accident had happened at exactly 8:20 P.M., and as much as she wanted to pretend there was nothing special about that time, the clock kept reminding her. She went into the dining room, where there were no clocks, and began working her way through the Sunday paper.

A few miles away, Maureen's parents and Ellen had spent much of the day with their own memories. These "milestone days," Louise told herself, were always the hardest. When the accident first happened, Maureen and her parents thought the passage of one year would begin to ease the pain. But the year was up, and it still hurt far more than they had even dreamed.

That night, neither Maureen nor her parents slept easily. Their thoughts were about Lisa, but also about the people who had received Lisa's eyes and kidneys. Today and tomorrow were milestones for them as well.

It was September, a year and a half since his cornea transplant, as Derrick Jackson walked up to the small reception window in the cornea-service waiting room of the Massachusetts Eye and Ear Infirmary. The waiting room was crowded, and Derrick looked at magazines and paced the halls to kill time.

Derrick was now living with Shirley, and their relationship continued to be a source of strength for both of them. Although he was still looking for a permanent job, he'd taken a couple of part-time jobs to help earn money. He had also remained faithful to his medical regimen. He put in his eye drops on schedule and had never missed a doctor's appointment.

187

But the biggest change was inside of him. Derrick was reaching out to people. He was no longer a loner. He had prayed for many people in his church who had been ill or troubled. He often went to their home to pray at their side. And this summer, after Shirley's older son, Charles, had tried out for a baseball team but been cut by the coach, Derrick stepped in. He persuaded two of his friends from church to join him, and together they organized a team for the boys who hadn't made the other one and found teams willing to play them. Charles, the quietest of Shirley's three children, and perhaps the most hurt by her divorce, looked up to Derrick and related to him as he would to a father.

After an hour's wait, Derrick was led into Dr. Kenyon's office.

"Let's start with the eye chart," Kenyon said.

He began with letters in the middle of the chart.

"Which way is this pointing?" Kenyon asked.

"That way," Derrick said, pointing in the correct direction. Kenyon moved down to near the bottom of the letters chart, and Derrick still got the correct answers.

Then he handed Derrick a card with very fine print on it. Derrick took his time. He read it slowly, but he read it.

"Amazing," Kenyon said, "just amazing. Your vision in the right eye is twenty–twenty-five. That's better than most of the people walking around on the street out there."

Kenyon tested the interoccular pressure by pressing a tonometer against Derrick's cornea. It was normal.

Kenyon palpated around the eye and then examined it through a slit lamp, which magnified his view. As Kenyon looked, he saw the eyeball vibrate noticeably, but he was not alarmed. It was a condition called nystagmus, common to people whose vision has been impaired. It causes them to lose the ability to focus their eye steadily. It was likely never to go away, but it did not appreciably interfere with Derrick's sight. Kenyon also checked over the area where he'd put in the corneal stitches. It was clear and clean, no sign of infection.

Kenyon drew aw y from the slit lamp and leaned back in his chair. "In my more than ten years of performing cornea transplants," he told Derrick, "this is the best one I've ever seen. This is a perfect cornea transplant."

Jo Leslie headed down a brightly lit corridor of the rehab unit at Shocktrauma. Every time she'd walked these corridors before, it seemed she'd been in a hurry to console a family, evaluate a donor, or check on test results. But now, as she moved through the cluttered halls on a September afternoon, eighteen months after procuring Lisa Kelly's organs, she walked more leisurely.

The corridor smelled of cleaning fluid mixed with the sharp scents of medications and antiseptic. It was a distinctive hospital odor that had always been a part of her professional life.

She looked at the patients. Some rested quietly in their rooms, others walked the halls. Most were near recovery and would soon be discharged. Even though virtually every patient brought to Shocktrauma was critically injured, a few had been so badly hurt when they arrived that Jo had immediately evaluated them as potential donors. She recognized some of them.

As she passed the nurses' station, Jo glanced at _miliar faces of doctors and nurses. Today she was more aware than usual of the many dramas that take place in the hospital, more in one day than most people experience in a lifetime. Then it hit her: *I won't be part of this anymore.* She had routinely dealt with people's losses, but now she had to deal with her own.

After directing Maryland's organ-procurement program for two years, and spending more than five years in a field that had consumed her, Jo was leaving. The decision, made that afternoon, was irrevocable. Soon she would begin teaching others what she had learned about dealing with donor families and procuring human organs in her new position with the Medical Eye Bank. In the past, that institution usually had relied on physicians to gain family permission to procure corneas. Now, Jo would specially train the Eye Bank personnel to deal with and support donor families. She also was planning to increase her number of speaking engagements — to continue to proselytize on organ transplantation around the country.

Back at her office, Jo slipped off her lab coat for the last time and within a half hour was driving along Pratt Street on her way home.

It was a balmy summer afternoon, and Jo rolled down her windows and felt the sun pour into her VW bus. At a stoplight, Jo threw back her head and closed her eyes. She took a long, deep breath that was almost a sigh. The light changed, but Jo just sat there with her eyes closed, allowing the sun to bathe her with its warmth. This, she said to herself, is the most relaxed I've felt in six months.

She and Rick had remained together, but Jo wanted to be closer, to spend more time with him. They'd gone on a week's vacation to New England during the summer. They enjoyed quiet dinners and reading on the beach. "I feel like I've died and gone to heaven," she'd told him. She'd dreaded going back to her office and at the same time felt guilty about being away.

This was a symptom of her growing ambivalence toward her work, which was expressed in other ways as well. One night, sitting on her back porch having drinks with Fran Danella after an exhausting day, Jo had said, "I've got to get out of the trenches, but I'm so afraid of losing something important."

She meant how important her work was to her. She feared that she'd miss the intensely human experiences she faced in organ procurement. She loved her work and she hated it, but maybe mostly she needed it. As painful as donor experiences often were, Jo was moved and drawn to them.

She had recently dealt with the father of a beautiful young woman who'd suffered brain death from a massive stroke. On the other side of the waiting room was the girl's boyfriend, who, Jo learned, had not spoken to the father since a bitter split several months earlier.

Jo had approached the father, but was really speaking to both of them. "I can't begin to know how terrible this is for you," she said, "and I want to tell you how sorry I am for what's happened. I'd like to ask you if you would consider donating your daughter's organs."

Both men looked searchingly at Jo, and then at each other. "If you want to talk it over," Jo said, "I'll be here to answer any questions."

The men talked to one another for a few minutes. Then they both dissolved into tears, and embraced.

"We'd like to donate," the father said, and Jo felt that she'd played some small part in their reconciliation. It was moments like these that she feared she'd never be a part of again.

In deciding to leave, there had been another problem. Jo no longer believed she could do the kind of job she wanted, or build the kind of organ-procurement network she'd envisioned.

After the Cumberland incident the previous November, when the on-call surgeon had refused to go with her to procure kidneys, Jo had realized that others were not as committed as she and her staff were to procuring donor organs. Whenever she'd talked about that incident, she'd pointed to it as one of the most disillusioning experiences in her life.

It had been compounded in her mind by a similar incident. A young man badly injured in an auto accident had been brought into Shocktrauma. He remained alive for several hours, but died before a surgeon could be located to remove his kidneys. The on-call surgeon had gone to his vacation home and apparently had not notified Jo's office. The result was that two potential recipients were left without kidneys, and the young man's parents, who had wished their son to become a donor, were left without that small consolation.

Jo realized it was naïve to say she had become disillusioned. She knew medicine had other priorities than her own. She also knew transplant surgeons always did other kinds of surgery as well, and that transplants were often not their major medical concern. But in the things that mattered to her, Jo saw the world in black and white terms. And because little mattered to her more than her work, she had little room for compromise.

She'd also been badly disappointed when her plan to merge the Medical Eye Bank and her own center into one organ-procurement program had been scuttled. She had negotiated with the Eye Bank directors since February, and they had endorsed the idea. She'd also met with the representatives of the three Baltimore hospitals that oversaw her center. She'd told them the merger would create the best organ-procurement center in the country.

For Jo, this would have been the culmination of her own ambition and would represent a major, important step in organ procurement. She'd promoted her vision for weeks, but after a series of formal presentations in May and June, the idea began to lose steam. Although different explanations were offered, it came down to one thing: politics.

Doctors at one of the hospitals feared the Medical Eye Bank, which had an international reputation, would gain too much control. Others worried that it would make Johns Hopkins, one of the best hospitals in the country, even more famous.

After the merger proposal had fallen through for good in the early summer, Jo realized it was only a matter of time before she'd leave. When she mentioned this to one of the surgeons, he had strongly urged her to stay on.

"You're doing a great job," he'd told her. "Things will get better."

192

She'd thanked him, but said, "I'm not doing this job just to bring in a paycheck. I'm doing it for me and for my vision of what organ procurement could become. It's tough to see someone just stomp all over your dream."

Jo turned right onto East Baltimore Street and drove along the northern edge of Patterson Park. The park had always represented to her a source of serenity and normalcy. And as she drove past it, she wondered how she would react to her new life — to being "normal" herself. It's over, it's really over, she thought, and her two warring emotions — regret and relief — welled up within her again.

A few days later, Jo and Fran sat on Jo's back deck, talking. Though saddened at Jo's departure, Fran planned to stay on, at least for the immediate future.

Fran had been in organ procurement for a much shorter time than Jo, yet she'd already experienced many of the same emotional ups and downs. They'd both been encouraged that recently many of the doctors with whom they often worked recognized the difficulty of their job. Most, however, did not.

The week before, Fran had mentioned to one surgeon how hard it was to deal with the donor families. He'd responded by telling her that getting kidneys was her job, not helping donor families. "If you want to do that, you ought to be a social worker," he'd said. Fran was still angry over it.

Jo was reminded of an incident in which one of the surgeons chided her for accepting refusals from potential donor families. "Don't take no for an answer," he'd said. Approach it like a "selling job." "If it were me," the surgeon continued, "I'd tell the family that when the medical examiner performs the autopsy, he throws away the organs anyway. So why not put them to good use?"

"That's why my job is to get permissions, and yours isn't," Jo answered. The fact that over the past few months she'd increased her permission rate to more than 80 percent and had been thanked by countless families for her kindness was proof enough that she understood how to approach the families.

Fran's pager went off and Jo, conditioned after five years, jumped up and started for the phone. They looked at each other and laughed. "You know?" Jo said. "This is the first time in five years I haven't been attached to a pager. When I hear a beep, I've got to tell myself not to jump."

Fran came back from the phone. "That was Hopkins," she said. "There's a donor over there. I've got to go."

Jo walked her out to the car and waved as Fran drove away. "Don't let the bastards get you down," she shouted. Fran waved back.

Jo stood there for several minutes, absentmindedly scratching the back of her hand. Then she noticed something and held her hand up to examine it in the remaining sunlight: those perfusion-fluid splotches were nearly gone.

The next few months were happily uneventful for Matthew and his family. One day they received a call from Ron Dreffer, the Cincinnati organ-procurement coordinator who had delivered Lisa's kidney to Matthew, asking them to be a part of Organ Donation Awareness Week. The week's highlight was a reception at the Westin Hotel. Many attended, including people directly involved in organ procurement, as well as critical-care nurses and others to whom Dreffer wanted to direct his message.

To show what organ donation was all about, Dreffer invited a number of donor families and recipients to speak. On a small stage in one of the conference rooms, donor families told how their decision to donate had helped ease the pain of their loss. Recipients also spoke. A young mother whose baby daughter had received a liver transplant held her in front of everyone and said, "This is my speech right here." Another speaker was a twenty-year-old man who'd lived with a "new" kidney for sixteen years.

The Landises had also been invited to speak. Jim and Betty were nervous about speaking before so many people, but Jim said, "If it will help, I'll talk to anyone."

When they'd first arrived at the reception, people who hadn't seen Matthew for a while were astonished at how good he looked, and how much he'd grown.

When it was their turn to speak, Jim approached the microphone. He asked the audience's indulgence because he was so nervous. Then he spoke of Matthew's struggle and triumph.

"We've watched him grow day by day. We've also watched him play to exhaustion in the backyard, sometimes beyond exhaustion. And we've wondered sometimes whether he'd wake up or not.

"Matthew has a great vitality. It's been a fight for life, but he could never have had that fight without an organ donor. I'm sure you've seen a lot of failure and sadness in your work, and it takes courage to go on. But I want you to know that your caring and concern make a difference. Please gain strength from the fact that Matthew is alive, and well, and with you tonight."

PART III

TODAY

C arolyn Blanchard and her family still live in their California home. She continues on CAPD, and despite some infections at the dialysis access site — a common risk for CAPD patients — she remains healthy and active. Her husband, Tom, has fully recovered from the mysterious fatigue that plagued him and is involved in a rigorous exercise program. He's now working at an executive-level position with a defense contractor. Greg, nineteen, joined the California Conservation Corps. He is studying forestry and is out of doors most of the time, which he always loved. Linda was accepted at the University of California at Santa Cruz, where she is now a freshman.

Carolyn is working part-time as a secretary and has no plans to attempt another kidney transplant anytime in the near future. She'd hoped there would be a major breakthrough in organ transplantation, and thought at one time that Cyclosporine might be it. It was still an experimental drug at the time of her transplant, but is now regarded as one of the most important advances in organ transplantation.

Cyclosporine interrupts the message that is sent by the cells in the body's immune system to the cells that attack a "foreign body" — i.e., the transplanted organ. Rejection is moderated because the immune system doesn't realize a foreign body is there.

There are problems with Cyclosporine, the most significant one being that it can adversely affect the kidneys, which in some people prevents its use in kidney transplantation. Blood pressure is also higher in some transplant patients who have received Cyclosporine.

Another factor in Carolyn's decision to at least postpone another transplant is the improved quality of life she now enjoys on CAPD. Because it only takes a few minutes four times a day, instead of several hours three times a week as did hemodialysis, she not only has much more freedom, but her energy is also much greater.

She has no regrets about her decision to try a kidney transplant and feels that it helped her and her family through a difficult time in their lives.

"I still think of my donor family and hope life is treating them kindly," she says.

Kenneth Walsh lives in the same comfortable rooming house outside Boston that he's lived in for the past few years. The sight in his right eye, which received Lisa's cornea, has not improved much, although the cornea remains perfectly clear. "It's like having a Mercedes in the garage and no gas to run it," he says. His sight remains a small pinhole amid the darkness. About four months after receiving Lisa's cornea, he received another transplant in his left eye, but in ten months it had been rejected. He then received yet another cornea in that eye, and despite a couple of rejection episodes, it has remained clear enough for him to read again, aided by thick glasses, but without the need for a magnifying glass. Now past seventy, he hopes it will last as long as he does.

He continues to visit his relatives and goes up to New Hampshire with his brother and sister-in-law to play bingo. His attitude remains unchanged. "You take what life gives you," he says. "No use complaining about it."

Derrick Jackson's life has changed greatly. Two years after his transplant, he went on a week-long religious retreat in the Berkshire Mountains. When he returned, he told Shirley the Lord had told him he would soon begin a new phase of his life.

Soon after, Derrick was "called" to a new church in Chicopee, about ten miles from Springfield. It was an important test of his faith, because he didn't want to leave Shirley, nor did she want him to. They remained in frequent phone contact, and Shirley often drove to Chicopee to see him, but the separation was painful for both of them.

After a few months, he was "called" back to Springfield. Derrick and Shirley were married later that year. Derrick was recently hired by the Springfield post office in a custodial position. It's his first full-time job ever, and he's extremely happy to have it. The cornea he received from Lisa remains perfect.

Derrick continues to help with Shirley's children. He participates with the boys in Royal Rangers, a scouting and Bible study program sponsored by their church. Elizabeth continues to be an outstanding student, and Derrick recently helped her rehearse her part for a school play.

"I've been given a lot," he says, "I'd like to give a few things back."

It was Sunday morning. High clouds blocked the sun, but it was still unusually warm for mid-April. As the Washington suburbs disappeared along Route Seventy, and the Maryland countryside began, Jim remarked to Betty how similar it was to Ohio. They were all dressed in their Sunday best. Matthew wore gray slacks and a bright red blazer that Betty's mother had sewn, and Betty and the girls were in dresses. Jim sat next to Matthew in the front seat of the car, and Matthew pretended to fall off to sleep. Jim touched him on the forehead, and Matthew opened his eyes.

"I'm not asleep," he laughed.

"You sure looked like it, Bubby," Jim said.

What Jim and Betty had wanted to do — but which had always seemed impossible — was now about to happen. They were on their way to meet the Kellys, the first such meeting in Jo Leslie's experience. A few months earlier, when Jo, who had been involved in training organ-procurement coordinators, first had learned that they wanted to meet, she'd reconsidered the reasons why such meetings were strongly discouraged. Matthew's kidney was functioning beautifully. Also, he was more than three years post-transplant and out of danger. This eliminated Jo's major worry that the Kellys would grieve twice. Jo also knew how anxious the families were to meet, and she was also anxious to meet them. So, having once united them in spirit, she helped unite them in body.

As Jim and Betty neared the rendezvous point, where they would meet Jo and her new husband, Rick Gjesdal, and then go to the Kellys', their anticipation grew. Will they like us? Betty wondered to herself. Will seeing Matthew give them a lift, or will it be a hard reminder of the daughter they lost? She sat quietly and thought.

"Are we there yet?" Matthew asked several times.

"Not yet," Jim answered. "Just a little farther."

A few miles later, they approached an intersection, and Jim looked across the street.

"There's the BP gas station," he said. "I guess we're here."

In a few minutes, Jo's yellow VW bus arrived at the station. Jo and Rick, who had met the Landises when they first arrived two days earlier, got out of their bus to greet Jim, Betty, and the children. Maureen was called at about 10:30 and told everyone had arrived.

"Give me ten minutes to get there," she said. Her voice was excited.

Maureen immediately called her mother.

"They're here," she said. "I'm going to get them now. See you in twenty minutes."

As she made the five-mile drive from her home to the gas station, her nervousness increased. She'd thought about this meeting for months, and what it would be like to see the little boy in whom part of Lisa still lived.

As she drove into the gas station, Maureen saw Matthew for the first time. She stopped her car and got out. Matthew walked toward her. She hadn't been prepared to see a little boy who looked so healthy, or attractive.

"A redhead," she yelled. She dropped to her knees and held out her arms, and he walked right to her. She wrapped her arms around his sturdy shoulders. "He's so beautiful," she said. Matthew smiled, but seemed a little perplexed that this total stranger was so affectionate.

Then Maureen stood and moved toward Jim and Betty.

Jim extended his hand and said, "Hi, I'm . . ."

He never got the words out. Maureen ignored his outstretched hand, and they moved toward one another as if they'd been close friends for years. Their embrace was immediate. Maureen and Jo hugged, and then Maureen turned to Betty, who had stood off to the side. These two young women, both about the same age, moved toward one another wordlessly and stood together in the parking lot, with their arms wrapped around one another.

Maureen hugged Janie and Valerie, then walked to her Bronco to lead the short drive to her parents' home.

"Anyone want to come with me?" she asked.

Betty took Matthew's hand, and they hopped into the back of Maureen's car. Jim and the girls, and Jo and Rick, followed in this small caravan. Maureen pulled out of the gas station parking lot and glanced back at the intersection.

"That's where Lisa's accident happened," she said calmly. "I didn't know if you knew." Betty looked back at the traffic light and the small group of nearby stores and nodded silently.

Maureen drove on the two-lane road for little more than two miles, then made a right turn onto a winding, narrow road that led to her parents' home.

"It's so pretty and peaceful out here," Betty said.

"When Dad moved us out here I must have hated him for a year. I just couldn't stand the place. There was no one else out here then. Of course, I came to love it," she said.

Matthew sat quietly absorbing everything.

Maureen turned to look at Betty and Matthew. "You're gonna see kids coming out of the woodwork when we get there. My folks have two young foster brothers now, Buster and Ellis. And I mean to tell you, Buster's really something. I'm hoping my brother Don's there. He's got a boy about your age, Matthew."

After a mile along this narrow road, Maureen took a sharp right onto a gravel driveway that led to the Kelly home. Trees were budding in the front yard, and young children were scampering outside.

They all left their cars and walked along the gravel path. Jo went over to Matthew, who was standing next to Maureen.

Maureen still appeared nervous. "Mom is anxious to see this little guy. I'd better take him in to meet her," she said.

Maureen opened the front door and walked through the small, neat living room toward the kitchen, where her mother was preparing the lunch.

Louise Kelly stepped into the living room. She seemed transfixed by Matthew, who stood shyly in front of her and stared at her with his curious brown eyes. As Maureen tried to say Matthew's name, her voice broke, and both she and her mother held on to one another and wept openly.

Jo was in a chair near the door and reached for Matthew's

hand. He sat silently next to her on the chair. For several moments not a word was spoken, and then Jim, Janie, and Rick all came into the house, and Maureen and Louise brushed away their tears as people found places to sit down.

Debbie, the foster child the Kellys had adopted soon after Lisa's death, and who bore a physical and temperamental resemblance to Lisa, came downstairs into the living room. She glanced over at Janie, who was about her age, and asked her if she wanted to come upstairs and play with her. Janie leapt at the chance to leave a room full of adults. Eugene Kelly, wearing a white shirt and dark suspenders, came in from outdoors and stood at the far end of the living room and looked directly at Matthew for a long time, but said nothing. He sat down in an easy chair near Louise; Tom, the Kellys' youngest natural child, sat on the other side of his mother. Now twenty-four, and wearing a beard, he was accompanied by his wife, Carla, who was pregnant with their first child.

As they all settled in their seats, a sense of the moment seemed to inhibit conversation. It was broken when Maureen stood up and walked over to the fireplace mantel, and took down the high school picture of Lisa, which had occupied the same spot for the past four years. She passed it over to Jim and Betty.

They studied Lisa's face, with its delicate features, and the long waves of blond hair. They both shook their heads, as if Lisa's loss was suddenly made real to them. Betty looked up at Louise and said, "She was so beautiful."

"Yes, she was. And on the inside, too," Louise said.

Then Maureen began passing around more photographs that she'd kept in a box.

"We thought you might like to see what Lisa was like," she said.

"Yes, we want to," Betty answered.

The photos were a record of Lisa's short life. Here she was

at three. Here at the beach. Another on horseback, and one of her in her Sunday best. And another taken shortly before she was killed.

Matthew studied each one. He knew that the pictures he was looking at were the girl who had given him his kidney, but he said nothing. Jim turned toward Louise and said in a soft voice, "He understands why he's here, but I'm not sure at his age how much he appreciates it." Louise nodded.

Maureen held one photograph up in front of her. "This is my favorite. Lisa was only about four then."

It showed Lisa, her hair platinum blond, smiling on Eugene Kelly's lap.

"I'm gonna get that one restored and framed," Maureen said.

Others soon joined the group. Maureen's brother, Don, two years younger than she, entered the room. Maureen was happy he was there, and also a little surprised. He still hadn't openly spoken about Lisa since the night more than three years earlier when he'd smashed his fist against the brick wall of the hospital after he'd first learned she'd been killed. He was of medium height with a slender, muscular build and had the hands of a man who worked with them. He wore a shirt open at the collar and sat quietly in the corner, preferring to observe instead of participate. Next to him was his wife, Gwen, a lively blond woman. She was as effusive as he was quiet. Their son, Danny, eight, bounded into the living room. His face was flushed with color and he had an excited look in his eye.

"Wanna come outside with me?" he hollered to Matthew.

Matthew looked at Betty, who gave her approval, and he took off his red blazer and darted out the front door with Danny.

After the boys were out of the house, Gwen, Danny's mother, remarked, "He talked about Lisa all the way over here today. He said, 'It's nice that Lisa gave Matthew her kidney, so he could live.' "

As the two families grew more familiar with one another,

206

their nervousness eased and conversation became more informal and relaxed. To Jo, it began to look and sound like a normal family dinner on Sunday afternoon.

Jo asked if Ellen, Lisa's blood sister, would be joining them. Louise explained she was working this day, but said the real reason was her continuing difficulty with her sister's death.

"They were this close," Louise said, holding up two entwined fingers. "She'll talk about the good times, but she hates to be reminded of the bad times. She didn't think she could hold up today."

"My dad's quiet about it too," Maureen said when her father was out of the room briefly. "I think one way he deals with it is the chickens. Before she died, Lisa told him, 'Dad, when you retire, we'll raise chickens in the backyard . . .' " Maureen's voice broke for a moment. "Now he's got five chickens out there."

Maureen was sitting on the stairs, overlooking the living room. Eugene came back into the living room and sat next to Louise again. Maureen looked over at him, and then directly at Jim and Betty. "I thank God my father had the courage to say yes to Jo that night. I didn't have it — I was hurting so bad. I just wanted her back, even though I knew she was gone. I was holding on to that thread of hope that some miracle would bring her back. . . . I wanted you two to know that."

In the middle of her story, her brother Don had left the room.

Louise turned to Jo Leslie and spoke almost in a whisper. "They didn't tell me that night about the organ donation, and I'm glad they didn't. I don't think I would have been able to handle it then."

The mood of sadness was shattered by Matthew charging through the front door into the living room.

"Please gimme the car keys," he shouted to Jim. "I want to put on my jeans."

Jim handed Matthew the keys.

207

"Don't give them to Danny," Eugene called out. "He's liable to drive."

"How many foster kids have you all had over the years?" Jo asked.

Someone guessed twenty-five. "More than that," Louise said. "I lost count, but it must be at least thirty or forty by now."

Louise said their present foster children, Buster and his brother, had come a few months earlier, both badly abused, much like Lisa had been seventeen years earlier. "Buster's teeth were just about all gone," she said. "First thing I did was to take him to Sinai Hospital in Baltimore to get him looked at. They put him under full anesthesia and worked on him nine hours, and his teeth are doing real fine, now."

Someone suggested they all walk outside to take pictures of one another, and they all congregated on the Kellys' front lawn that overlooked a wide expanse of open land. The little boys, Matthew, Danny, Buster, and his brother Ellis, heard the commotion and came from the backyard.

Matthew eyed a gnarled old tree in the front yard and shimmied up to the lowest limb. Eugene came over and helped him.

"You got it now?" Eugene asked.

"Yep, I got it," Matthew answered triumphantly as he stood on the limb. Danny climbed up to join him and they stood together with their arms around one another.

"Where'd Matthew get that red hair from?" Maureen asked.

"Jim's grandmother was a redhead," Betty told her. "I'm adopted, so I'm not sure about my side of the family."

The little boys all ran out back again, and Eugene and Jo followed. Buster pounded a baseball bat on the dirt pile, and Matthew and Danny climbed another tree together. When they came down, Eugene pushed both of them on the swing for a few minutes. Then one of the boys opened up the toolshed to get something, and Jo peeked in and found it full of toys and kids' bikes.

"It looks like a toy store in there," she said.

"Yeah, there's no room for my tools in there," Eugene chuckled.

Jo and Eugene went back inside to join the others for lunch. Louise had prepared a spread of salads, roast beef, and turkey, along with cakes, fruit, and cookies for dessert. Eugene was on the stairs near Maureen and talked with Jo.

"Lisa would just have been thrilled to see that little boy. She loved little kids," he said. Then he paused for a second and said, "Wherever she is, I think she knows."

As people sat around the living room eating lunch, the conversation shifted back and forth from one or two people talking to each other, to one person talking to the entire group. The tone of the conversation shifted too. Sometimes they laughed over family stories, sometimes they became emotional. The Kellys wanted to tell Jim and Betty what Lisa was like, as if to let them know that the kidney that kept Matthew alive was from a person they would have liked, even loved.

Louise told them how patient Lisa was, and how much she loved children. "She was just so gentle to little kids. She was a good kid," she said, her voice trailing off.

"All the time I knew her," Maureen told Jim and Betty, "I can remember just one time seeing her get real mad. She and Ellen got to fighting. I mean they went toe to toe, and I turned to Mom and said, 'I've never seen Lisa get that mad.' And Mom said, 'Let 'em go. Ellen's just pushed her too far this time.'"

Jim and Betty laughed along with the others. However, when Lisa's name came up, Don had left the room again.

His wife, Gwen, nodded at his empty chair. "He still won't talk about her. If I mention Lisa's name he'll respond, but then he'll change the subject real fast."

In the kitchen, Don talked with his mother and Betty, who were there getting coffee. He was intensely interested in Matthew. He asked Betty how long the kidney might last and what medications he had to take.

"The doctors say the kidney could last indefinitely," she told him. "Everything about Matthew right now is normal. He's only on two medications, and the doctors say his immune system is very close to normal. He shouldn't be any more susceptible to colds and other infections than anyone else."

Don appeared pleased to hear it. "He looks real strong and healthy," he said.

"He is, thanks to what your family did for him," Betty said.

Don nodded his head, but said nothing more.

"He is a whirlwind," someone remarked of Matthew.

Jim told them that two years after the kidney transplant, Matthew was operated on to straighten out his leg bones.

"He had what they call renal rickets, caused by his old kidney problem, which in turn prevented him from absorbing vitamin D properly. It caused his leg bones to bow. So, if he put his knees together, he couldn't get his ankles closer than fourteen inches apart. They had to break his bones and reset them. So he got around for a few weeks lugging his body cast. The day he was scheduled to go back to the hospital to have it cut off, Betty and I woke up very early in the morning and heard a pounding noise. I got up and began looking around, and I found Matthew in the garage, sitting on the floor, banging his cast off with a hammer. Chunks of it were lying all around. The doctors told him he'd be out of the cast that day, and he was making sure he would be."

"I'll bet that kind of spirit is why he's alive," Maureen said admiringly.

"He's got plenty of fight, I can assure you of that," Jim said.

Eugene quietly stood up and walked out to the backyard again. The four boys were now busily playing in the dirt pile. Buster picked up the bat and started pounding the dirt again, near the other boys.

"Buster, I don't think you ought to do that," Eugene said in a steady voice.

Buster looked over at him and dropped the bat.

Matthew approached Eugene and sat next to him on the picnic table bench.

"How many chickens do you have?" he asked.

"I got five of them. You want to look at them?" Eugene asked.

"Yeah," Matthew answered.

Eugene took his hand, and they walked across the yard to the chicken coop he'd built. Matthew watched with fascination as the chickens pecked away at the tiny bits of food left on the ground.

For several moments, the two of them stood silently, hand in hand, watching the chickens. Then they both turned slowly, and Eugene looked at Matthew and said, "Want me to push you on the swing again?"

Matthew said he did, and they walked over to the swings. Danny sat on the swing next to him, and Eugene, now over sixty, stood and pushed the swings until the boys wanted to do something else.

Inside the house, Jim glanced at his watch and knew it was nearing the time to leave. They had to catch a plane back to Cincinnati late that afternoon. Everyone seemed reluctant to part, but slowly they stood up and walked outside to the front lawn. They had been together less than four hours. Matthew, Danny, Buster, and Ellis all appeared. Matthew had dirt stains on his knees. Addresses were exchanged between the families, and they all promised to write and send pictures.

Jim stood on the front steps and extended his hand to Eugene. "Thank you for your hospitality, and thank you for everything else you've done for us."

Eugene began to say, "We're very happy to have . . . ," but

he couldn't finish, and Jim nodded, patted him on the back, and the fathers bade each other goodbye.

Tom, standing next to his wife, Carla, shook Jim's hand and told him he was glad they came, that it was a wonderful day for his family. Gwen threw her arms around everyone and thanked them all; so did Valerie and Janie.

Betty and Maureen embraced again; so did Jim and Louise. The embraces were strong and long, and tears came spontaneously to everyone's eyes. It was as if by holding and sharing, they all were helping erase many hard memories and replace them with newer, happier ones.

"Thank you for coming. This has meant so much to us," Maureen told Jim.

"To us too," Jim said.

Almost lost among the adults were the small figures of Matthew and Danny. They had their arms wrapped around one another, and then they turned and patted each other on the back.

"You're my friend," Danny said.

"You're my friend, too," Matthew answered. "You come to my house and play next time."

Jo stood and watched them, and then looked over at Don, Danny's father. He stared at the two boys, and his face was a portrait of joy. Then his eyes misted, and Jo saw a trace of sadness in them.

Matthew ran up to Jo, threw his arms around her neck, gave her a strong hug, and said, "We're leaving, I just wanted to tell you goodbye."

Jo hugged him back and told him, "I love you bunches."

Then, from the edge of the yard, Don moved toward Jim, who was nearing the car. Don held Jim's arm tightly and said in an emotional voice, "Take care of that little boy of yours for us."

Jim looked at him and said, "I will."

Don nodded and walked away.

Maureen and her mother stood in the middle of the lawn as the sun broke through the clouds, and the gathering slowly dispersed. They watched Matthew giggling and laughing and, in a last flurry of activity, run up and hug Eugene. Then he ran to Louise and Maureen and gave them one final hug and kiss.

"You come see us again," Louise told him.

"Okay, you come to our house, too," he said.

As Maureen watched Matthew walk toward the waiting car, she thought to herself, You can't tell me God has stopped making miracles.

Finally, the goodbyes were over, and the two families parted.

As Jo and Rick drove home toward Baltimore, she asked him what he thought. His eyes misted as he spoke.

"Those families have gone through so much . . . and they both had so much love and laughter," he said.

"I know," Jo said. "I'm so glad they got together. I don't really see why we should have rules against these meetings, as long as the recipients and donor families want them. I don't think we have to protect them from grieving twice. I think the donor families can tolerate that, because I think it's a lot better for them to have this kind of opportunity. I sure think it would help heal a lot of anger and hurt."

Jo was entering the University of Maryland in the summer to begin a three-year program in clinical psychology. She planned to concentrate on death and dying, and she already knew her thesis would be on donor families. The experience she'd witnessed this day would be part of that, and part of her growing vision to help people cope with this hardest of life's realities.

During the drive to the airport, Betty said she felt such love and communion at the Kelly house she was overwhelmed by it. "They seem like my family. It was as if I'd always known them," she told Jim.

Valerie, who'd sat quietly for most of the meeting, wept during much of the hour-long drive. When Betty asked her why she was crying, she answered, "Everything."

Matthew barely said a word for the entire drive, and Janie slept.

"There was a purpose in it for me," Jim said. "Seeing all the love in that family gave a lot to me. I just hope we were able to give something back to them. They're a wonderful family."

With the guests gone, Maureen remained at her parents' home to help her mother clean up. After the last dish was dried and the extra food wrapped and put away in the refrigerator, the Kellys sat in the living room. They talked of how much they liked Jim and Betty and their family. They'd found them warm and down to earth. "Real solid people," Louise said.

"It gave me such a lift to see Matthew," Maureen said. "I expected to see a sickly little boy. But he was so healthy I couldn't believe it."

"And so affectionate," Louise added.

The day stirred many emotions for them, but the strongest was their feeling that they had been a part of something that was starting a new phase of healing. They would share these feelings with Ellen, and hope it would ease her burden.

Maureen leaned back in her chair. Part of her was sobbing, another part laughing at the joyous memories of that day. She reflected for a moment and said, "You know, for the first time since Lisa's death, I'm finally at peace with it."

Louise looked over at her and in a soft voice said, "So am I."